The Family Squeeze

Surviving the Sandwich Generation

'The Sandwich Generation' refers to the growing number of middle-aged people who must care for both children and elderly parents while trying to manage the stress of full-time jobs. Advances in technology and medicine are helping us to live longer – but not without extended care from our families. At the same time, the economic climate is making it difficult for young adults to leave home and start their own lives; they are often 'boomeranged' back to their parents for financial help, emotional support, and accommodation.

In *The Family Squeeze*, Suzanne Kingsmill and Ben Schlesinger trace the day-to-day life of a typical family caught up in this situation. They guide the reader through various scenarios, paying particular attention to the 'woman in the middle,' who has traditionally been the caregiver to young and old but is now also a full-time member of the workforce. Each scenario is followed by comments, advice, and suggestions that will help the reader understand each stage of the game. The resource section includes an extensive annotated bibliography, as well as a list of selected services in Canada and the United States. Internet resources are also listed.

Any person who is, or about to become, a member of the Sandwich Generation will find this a helpful guide for coping with the conflicting demands of family and work.

SUZANNE KINGSMILL is the author of two popular books and numerous articles which have appeared in major periodicals around the world.

BENJAMIN SCHLESINGER is Professor Emeritus in the Faculty of Social Work at the University of Toronto. He has previously published 22 academic books.

The Family Squeeze

Surviving the Sandwich Generation

Suzanne Kingsmill and Benjamin Schlesinger

UNIVERSITY OF TORONTO PRESS
Toronto Buffalo London

ISBN 0-8020-0764-3 (cloth)
ISBN 0-8020-7134-1 (paper)

Printed on acid-free paper

Canadian Cataloguing in Publication Data

Kingsmill, Suzanne
    The family squeeze : surviving the sandwich generation

    Includes bibliographical references and index.
    ISBN 0-8020-0764-3 (bound)   ISBN 0-8020-7134-1 (pbk.)

    1. Sandwich generation   2. Middle aged women – Family relationships.
    I. Schlesinger. Benjamin, 1928–   .   II. Title.

    HQ1059.4 K56 1998   306.874   C98-930756-5

University of Toronto Press acknowledges the financial assistance to its
publishing program of the Canada Council for the Arts and the Ontario Arts
Council.

Contents

Peter and David feel the three-generation pinch as Grandma comes home from hospital.
Three generations living under one roof – the pros and cons

Rebecca gets bawled out at work for taking time off to help her family.
Are there resources available at work? ~ What employers can do to help ~ How the new conservatism is undermining the ability of soucieres to care ~ Are there resources available for the souciere?

It's too much and Rebecca's parents plan to move to a retirement home.
Where can elders move once they leave their homes or families? ~ How to choose retirement homes/homes for the aged/nursing homes ~ Coping with guilt

Rebecca learns her mother knows nothing about finances and is fearful of what will happen if she outlives her husband.
Widowhood and how to deal with it ~ Planning ahead – Financial planning for old age

Preface

If you are feeling the effects of the 'family squeeze,' with demands from your children coming at you from one direction, the increasing needs of your aging parents pulling at you from another, and your job beckoning daily, then welcome to the Sandwich Generation. If you're not being squeezed at the moment, welcome anyway, because it's only a matter of time before you will be.

The strict definition of the Sandwich Generation, a term coined by Dorothy Miller in 1981,[1] is anyone around the age of 52 who has aging parents who require help and who at the same time has at least one adult child who has returned to live at home. This definition has been broadened in recent years to include younger children who have not yet left home. Whatever the definition, almost all of us are going to find ourselves in a sandwich at some point in our lives. This book will address the problems of those 'women in the middle' who are married and have elderly parents and adult children who have returned home. Many of the problems they face are similar to those of women whose children have not yet left home.

Thanks to modern technology, more and more people are living longer and longer. At the same time, fewer children are being born who might help care for the elderly. Fertility rates have been dropping steadily; also, more women are having children later in life, which increases the likelihood that they will be caught in the sandwich. At the same time, adult children are returning home – or never leaving it – because of unemployment, marriage breakdown, and educational or financial needs. When you add to all this the fact that more and more women are working full time where once they stayed home and provided care for the young and old, you have the potential for a host of problems in the largely uncharted waters navigated by the Sandwich Generations.

And even if you're only being pushed from one side with aging parents, or from the other with teenage or adult kids, read on. This book is for all of you caregivers (most of whom are women) who are struggling to find time to do it all while facing your own mortality, even as you see that mortality staring back in the faces of your parents (and altogether missing in the recklessness of your kids). It's for all of you who thought that your children would grow up, leave home, and live independent lives, and that your parents would never grow old. It's for all of you who have been looking forward to the day when you would be on your own once again, and able to do some of the things you always wanted, but are wondering now if that day will ever come. It's for those of you who are highly, or moderately, or slightly stressed by your caregiving duties; and for those of you who know that in caring for your parents and your children there will be times when the rewards are few, times when you can barely cope and will need help, times when life is OK and the rewards are many, times when the sandwich is good, and times when the sandwich makes you choke. You are the caregivers of yesterday, today, and tomorrow: the ones who will care for your children, your elderly parents, and one day your ailing spouses, in a caregiving career that spans a lifetime. You are the ones who need to learn how to spread the load of all that caregiving.

In each chapter, *The Family Squeeze* will walk you through the lives of a generic wife (Rebecca) and husband (Bryan) and their experience of being squeezed by their 14-year-old son Peter, 17-year-old daughter Danielle, and 21-year-old boomerang son David, and by Rebecca's parents. Comments, advice, and suggestions will follow each episode in the story that will help you understand and handle each stage of the game, whether it is mutually setting guidelines for your adult child or finding a retirement or nursing home for your parents.

Throughout this book we use the term 'souciaire' to mean an

informal caregiver, who is usually related to the care receiver; this is to differentiate between formal (i.e., paid) caregivers and informal (unpaid) *souciaires*. It is derived from the French word *souci*, meaning 'worry' or 'care.' It is used interchangeably with *caregiver* when we are talking of informal caregivers only.

We realize that we have covered only one aspect of the Sandwich Generation – namely, the 'family squeeze,' which involves young adult children living at home, elderly parents living in their own homes, and 'the woman in the middle.' We need further family studies to examine the following family situations:

- Families with small children.
- Families with institutionalized elderly.
- Families with elderly parents with Alzheimer's or other debilitating conditions.
- Ethnic families (i.e., how do they handle the sandwich family?).
- Males who do the caregiving in the sandwich family.

We have just begun to explore this emerging family pattern. As we near the twenty-first century we may find still other family issues facing the 'family squeeze.' What is surprising is that most families show great strength and resiliency in dealing with the Sandwich Generation.

The Family Squeeze

Surviving the Sandwich Generation

CHAPTER ONE

The Sandwich Generation

'Hi Mum, I'm home!' I stopped in my tracks. Without fail for a dozen years, every school day at 3:30, I had heard that line from each of our three kids. But I hadn't heard that particular voice saying those particular words for at least two years, because that particular son didn't live with us anymore.

David, at twenty-one, lived and worked on the other side of town; only our two youngest – Danielle, seventeen, and Peter, fourteen – were still at school and living at home. I dumped the newspapers and magazines I was lugging to the recycling bin onto the kitchen table and went to greet him, wondering why he had come in the front door. He never used that door, except on formal occasions. Bryan and I had drummed it into his head too many times as a kid that the front door and muddy shoes did not get along.

As I walked past our living room window I glanced outside and saw my father walking down the sidewalk to our house, peering curiously at David's two trunks, which were sprawled across our walkway. I suddenly remembered that I had promised to help him buy a birthday present for Mum on one of my rare days off work. He and Mum lived about twenty minutes away, and we'd agreed that he would get some exercise by walking over to pick me up. How could I have forgotten? Was I getting old? Surely not – at fifty-one I felt fit and in control of life as never before. My job at the library was rewarding and stimulating, and Bryan and I were hoping to plan our first mini-holiday alone in twenty years now that Danielle and Peter were old enough to look after themselves for a day or so – with a little guidance from my Mum, of course. It was to be a prelude to our soon-to-be-empty nest, a taste of all the good things to come – freedom after retirement and all that. No more responsibilities!

Dad would have to wait a few minutes, I thought, as I spied David standing in the front hall craning his neck as he looked into the kitchen, presumably looking for me. The front door stood wide open at his back as if he was unsure of his reception. He looked like a lost little boy, gripping a suitcase in either hand so tightly that his knuckles gleamed white. I felt all the old mothering instincts surging to the fore, those instincts that just seem to arise unbidden when a parent sees her child in trouble.

David looked awful. There were big circles under his deep, wide-set blue eyes. His usually shiny black hair was dull and lank and flopped over his eyes like a sheepdog's, and his jeans, which looked like they belonged to a much bigger version of himself, had huge rips in them. He hadn't shaved in several days, and his high cheek-bones jutted out so that they emphasized his sunken cheeks. He was wretchedly thin and looked as though he hadn't had a decent meal in weeks. He turned as he heard my footsteps on the polished wooden floor, his face pinched and nervous. I was trying to decide whether I should run up and hug him when he blurted out –

'They sacked me, Mum. Said they were downsizing and I was last hired so I'm first fired.'

The words struck me like a tidal wave – David had spent months searching for a computer programming job. I remembered our excitement when Astral Computer had offered him one that paid well and had long-term potential – or so we'd thought at the time.

'But David, they gave you a raise last month. How can they fire you?'

He shrugged. 'They can and they have.'

At that moment a horrible scream crashed into the house, as if to underscore my feelings. The silence that followed was unnerving. The sunlight streamed in through the open front door, and I saw the maple trees that lined the road swaying in the gentle spring breeze. David dropped his bags and half-turned as I moved past him and out onto the doorstep. I was aware of someone running down the sidewalk toward our bungalow, yelling something, but all I had eyes for was my eighty-one-year-old father lying sprawled over one of David's suitcases, gripping his right hip and writhing in pain.

The next few weeks were a blur for us. We ran ourselves ragged visiting my father in the hospital, helping my mother, trying to cheer up a depressed David as he moved back in with us, looking after Danielle and Peter, and putting in a full day's work. As Dad's broken hip slowly healed, things got easier, but it had been pretty intense for the first few weeks after he went home from the hospital. It had been too much for Mum, and I tried to help her as best I could while Dad slowly got back on his feet with the help of a walker.

With all the travelling to and from my parents' place, while juggling all my other obligations, I was exhausted emotionally and physically. I had forgotten there was a name for our plight until my next-door neighbour, Marje, blurted it out one day as I lay propped up on an outdoor lawnchair trying to snooze. She called it the Sandwich Generation.

'Sandwich Generation? What's that?' I asked as she watched me over the red picket fence we shared. I'd heard of the sandwich generation in passing, but I couldn't remember exactly what it was. I was only asking out of politeness. I couldn't just drop the hint that perhaps she might want to let me sleep – that would have been unneighbourly, and she'd done me a lot of favours over the years.

'Really, Rebecca, where have you been? The Sandwich Generation is all the middle-aged people who care for their elderly parents and their kids at the same time.' The reference to middle age hurt, but I tried to be nonchalant and pretend I wasn't alarmed at the thought that I was middle-aged. After all, I didn't *feel* middle-aged.

'So Bryan and I are supposed to be the filling in the middle?' I asked, grimacing at the thought of my son's gooey peanut-butter-and-honey sandwiches.

'That's right. The bottom layers of the sandwich are your kids, Danielle and Peter – and now David again too, because he's returned home and you're in essence looking after him. Right?'

'David's just home for a little while,' I protested. 'And he's looking after himself. He's an adult now.'

'Just because he's an adult doesn't mean he's looking after himself,' she said.

I had to admit she had a point.

'He cooks his own meals? Does his own laundry?' Marje was relentless. 'Boy, Rebecca, I don't ever remember you mentioning he did that when he lived at home.'

I squirmed in my chair. 'Well, he didn't exactly. I'm doing it for him now, but only for a while. There's no harm in that. He needs some time to get over losing his job so suddenly,' I added lamely. 'He says he won't be staying with us for too long.'

'Sure, Rebecca. In other words you're looking after him *indefinitely*.' Her emphasis on that last word made me feel uneasy, but she waved away my protests and continued: 'The top layer of the sandwich is your parents, or Bryan's parents, who are going to need more and more help as they get older.'

Bryan's parents? I hadn't even thought about them till now.

'You're the one who can help both slices,' Marje continued, unaware of my inner turmoil. 'There are all sorts of possible scenarios for a member of the Sandwich Generation. I have a friend whose mother is looking after her grandmother and her husband's mother at the same time, and she has two teenage kids and two adult kids living at home.'

'Don't tell me,' I said with a groan. 'A *club* sandwich?'

Marje smiled. 'Corny, eh? There are all kinds of different sandwich combos out there. It all depends on the make-up of the family – whether it's blended, single-parent, divorced, three, four, or five generations, poor, wealthy, or from different cultures and socioeconomic backgrounds ... it goes on and on. With all the different life scenarios, you can get really corny about the sandwich analogy – open-facers, butter-side down, double-decker, all dressed or plain. In other words, it's a real smorgasbord.'

I rolled my eyes at her analogy. Sandwiches and fixings and such were all well and good, but I couldn't get it out of my head that the purpose of a sandwich was to eat it. I wondered what that said about the Sandwich Generation.

'Of course, the analogy can bog down if you delve too deeply,' she added.

I couldn't have agreed more. I'd always thought of a sandwich as two outer slices *protecting* the innards, not squashing them. Few of us eat peanut butter straight from the jar – you need the bread to make it palatable. But as Marje was saying, the term Sandwich Generation had stuck.

Marje pressed on. 'The people in the middle can range in age from twenty to ninety, but most of them are like us – middle-aged and square in the middle between thirty-five and sixty-five, with adolescent or grown kids still living with us.'

'There can't be very many of us,' I said, wishing she'd stop rubbing in the middle-aged part.

'Wrong,' said Marje gleefully. 'There are almost three-and-a-half million of us in Canada (2). That's about ten per cent of the population, and that's just measured at one point in time. Of course, it's really a continuum. As fast as some of us leave the sandwich, many more – like you – are just entering it. For most of us the odds of being in a sandwich at some point are good. Anyone with parents and kids will likely be in and out of the sandwich more than once. And if it doesn't happen simultaneously, in a true sandwich, it will certainly happen sequentially – sometimes bumper to bumper as we raise our kids, then help our aging parents and finally our aging spouses. The one constant is that if we are part of a family, our caregiving days never end. The real question is what type of sandwich you're in.'

'How can you call it a *generation*?' I asked. I was a real stickler for semantics. 'It's not a generation at all if it includes twenty- and ninety-year-olds at the same time.'

'You're right, I guess,' Marje answered. She paused, grappling with her thoughts, before she continued –

'It spans many generations, and a person can move in and out of the sandwich more than once. Technically, it's not a developmental stage in our life cycle like menopause or puberty, since the Sandwich Generation, as you say, is made up of more than one generation. So strictly speaking it should be the Sandwich *Generations* (2). You know – plural? With an "s"?'

'How do you know so much about all this?' I asked.

'Because I've been the innards of a soggy double-decker for ten years, and you wouldn't believe the problems ...'

I didn't want to hear about it. The thought of what a soggy double-decker might involve (five generations all alive at one time?) was enough to scare me away. What I was wrestling with was that I really didn't believe there was much to the Sandwich Generation. I couldn't help but think that maybe the name was just the baby boomers' way of whining about things they didn't want to do. In other words, Sandwich Generations have always existed, so what's the problem?

Sure, I had to admit that it had been tough helping my parents while working full time, but it wasn't as though I could just ignore them in their time of need. Why did my responsibilities need a name, and what right did I have to complain any more than my parents or grandparents did? Sons and daughters have always cared for their parents and kids. Was it really any different than in the past? After all, three- and four-generation families have been with us for some time now, and families have looked after their children and their parents for generations. So what makes the Sandwich Generations of the late twentieth century any different from the Sandwich Generations of, say, fifty or a hundred or two hundred years ago?

*   *   *

Plenty, as Rebecca will soon find out first-hand, as her 'sandwich' unfolds in the following chapters. Times have changed. Rebecca is facing a different set of circumstances from those faced by her parents and grandparents – circumstances that have added a considerable burden not felt by past generations.

The Top Layer of the Sandwich Is Getting Older

We're living and lingering longer on this earth than at any other time in history. If Rebecca had been born in ancient Greece she likely would have been dead by 21. By 1900 she could have expected to live to be 49, and by 1980 her potential lifespan would have risen to 79 (2,3). Today, with an average life expectancy of about 74 for men and 80 for women, Rebecca can expect to live almost 60 years longer than her counterparts in ancient Greece.

For the first time in history, a fourth and even a fifth generation exists so that some families have three or four grandparents still alive and a couple of great-grandparents. This is the daunting double-decker of Marje's world.

Not so long ago we died young, from such things as tuberculosis, pneumonia, and typhoid. Today we have vaccines to stop major epidemics of diseases such as diphtheria, measles, and whooping cough. Smallpox has been eliminated, and we have antibiotics to deal with all manner of acute illnesses that used to prevent people from ever reaching old age. Deaths from infectious diseases have plummeted since 1900.

Our bodies are programmed to last only so long, no matter what medical wonders are invented. Instead of succumbing to acute illnesses as in the past, more and more of us are living long enough to experience chronic illnesses such as Alzheimer's, arthritis, diabetes, osteoporosis, and strokes. Chronic ailments such as these have replaced acute illnesses as the major health problems of the elderly. These ailments are incurable and ongoing and result in disability and dependency.

Caring for parents who are ill or who simply need 'a few chores done' is a given that none of us would question; but today caregivers or souciaires are providing more help – and more onerous help – to more people over more years than ever before. Our lifespans have lengthened to the point that we now find 65-year-olds looking after 85-year-olds. Ten per cent of people over 65 have a child over 65! In 1986, 11 per cent of Canadians, or about 2.7 million, were over 65 – up from 6 per cent in 1931. According to Statistics Canada, that figure now stands at 12 per cent. It will rise to 16 per cent by 2016 and to 25 per cent, or one in four Canadians, by 2041 (4, 5).

Statistics Canada also estimates that by 2041 the number of elderly 85 and older will have increased fivefold (5). The number of people more than a century old has tripled in the last twenty years and is expected to double again in another twenty. According to the Census, in 1991 there were 3,700 centenarians in Canada. This all adds up to more elderly in the population than ever before – and more years of caring for them. In 1900 we could expect to spend 9 years caring for our parents. Today we can expect to spend 18 years (6).

As baby boomers watch their parents age, interest in the elderly is increasing, and concern is rising as to who will look after them all when the time comes.

The Bottom Layer Is Shrinking

It's not an idle thought: at the same time as we are growing older, we are not replacing ourselves. Large families with seven and eight children were once the norm; nowadays couples are having far fewer children. The current fertility rate (less than 2 children per woman of childbearing age) is not enough to replace those who die. Smaller families means fewer children to care for aging parents; and with the increasingly transient nature of families, many children don't live anywhere near their aging parents. The caregivers of today are simply fewer than in the past; an 80-year-old of today has far fewer children to rely on than her mother did in her old age.

If it's a problem now, it stands to become worse as we baby boomers age, with fewer young than ever before to look after us in our old age, as fertility rates remain static. Baby boomers in Canada are some eight million strong, and by the time we are old we will represent the largest cohort of elderly ever seen on earth.

Statistics Canada estimates that the proportion of aged will rise more and more steeply as baby boomers reach old age; by 2041, the proportion of those under 18 – on whose backs our old age will ride – will have shrunk from today's 25 per cent to 19 per cent (5). With the workforce shrinking and the cohort of elderly growing at an accelerated pace, the problems of the Sandwich Generations will be greater in the future than they are now. Solutions must be found to ease today's burden so that tomorrow's will be less.

The Bottom Layer Is Sticking to the Home Like Velcro™

At the same time as the elderly population is increasing our children are having trouble extricating themselves from us and making it on their own. Ten years ago most of us expected to raise our children, educate them, and launch them into the world; after that point, we expected them to win their autonomy, pursue their own careers, and have families of their own, just as we had done several decades earlier. But we couldn't have predicted then that the economic climate would be so different now. Like so many others, Rebecca is facing a new trend, the extinction of the empty nest and the formation of the *cluttered* nest – something for which she is not prepared, either financially or emotionally.

In the past, leaving home was associated with marriage, employment, and education. In today's weakened economic climate, more and more young adults are delaying marriage and opting to remain at home to pursue the higher education they need to get a good job in a shrinking market. Others are returning home after failed marriages, or after losing their jobs in a world where job security is no longer a given, or after failing to cope financially in the world. With the housing crisis, the high cost of living, and rampant unemployment, they can save money by moving back. The 1991 census showed that most unmarried men and women aged 15 to 24 lived at home. Also, 33 per cent of unmarried women and 44 per cent of unmarried men aged 25 to 29 were living at home. Gone, it seems, are the days of the 1950s and 1960s when university-trained people had little difficulty finding work.

The Filling in the Sandwich: The Souciaires

The problem gets more complicated when we look at the souciaires. Time and time again, research shows that most caregivers of the young and old are women. More than 7 out of 10 people providing informal (read 'unpaid') care to the elderly are women, with daughters and daughters-in-law making up the largest group of sandwiched souciaires. Nearly 9 out of 10 women (89 per cent) will be souciaires of parents, or children, or both, at some time in their lives. More than 8 out of 10 (83 per cent) will care for children; nearly 4 out of 10 (37 per cent) will care for a disabled adult (6).

In the past, when most women did not work outside the home, it was assumed that they would look after the needs of both children and aging parents. But times have changed, and have brought new pressures. For the first time in history most women are working outside the home. In 1930 fewer than 1 in 4 women worked (24 per cent). Today, 8 out of 10 women work; together they make up nearly half the labour force (46 per cent) (3). Yet more than half of all working women also care for elderly relatives, and about 4 in every 10 women (40 per cent) are still raising children (7).

Because of the competing demands of caregiving and careers, which push many souciaires to saturation point, the informal, unpaid caregiving that people do has become more visible. Ironically, this is occurring at a time when a wave of conservatism is sweeping the country. As one result, families will certainly be called upon to play an ever larger role in caregiving. This is a cause for concern as times, unfortunately, have not changed where caregiving is concerned: women still do the lioness's share, even though most of them also work outside the home in an economic climate in which most families must have two incomes just to make ends meet. Men must be brought into the equation in a meaningful and equal way.

Caregiving duties are no less merely because a souciaire is working. Not surprisingly, the competing demands on our time are taking their toll. As sandwiched individuals, we may find ourselves limited emotionally, financially, and socially. Careers and marriages can suffer under the burden. Largely ignored by professional health care workers, we struggle to juggle parents, children, jobs, and leisure time, generally through trial and error. We often go on a wing and a prayer, hoping we are doing the right thing but often plagued by feelings of guilt, anger, and frustration.

In a world that expects women to care for their children and elderly parents but also says it's OK for them to work outside the home, how does someone like Rebecca reconcile the two without tearing herself apart? As it unfolds, the story of Rebecca and her family will illustrate all the joys and sorrows, problems and pluses, crises and solutions, that confront women and men of the Sandwich Generations.

CHAPTER TWO

Velcro™ Kids – The First Slice of the Sandwich

I pulled up in front of the house in my little rusty mini, let myself into the kitchen, and sighed with relief. It had taken a lot longer than I had thought to buy groceries for Mum and Dad, and I hoped Mum would soon get over the cold she'd picked up somewhere so that she could start shopping again. Dad still couldn't get out easily because of his walker. I grabbed some milk from the fridge and went into the living room, and jumped a mile. I hadn't expected anyone to be home, but there was David, all six feet of him, sprawled on the sofa leafing through a magazine and eating a bag of chips.

'Grandma called for you,' he said, glancing up at me. 'She can't find any butter in the groceries you bought and wanted to know if you could run some over later on.'

I looked at David and wondered why he couldn't have offered to do it, seeing as how he seemed to be doing nothing, but I didn't say anything. After all, they were *my* parents.

'I thought you were out job hunting,' I said, trying not to sound accusatory, but by the look on his face not succeeding very well.

He shrugged.

'What are you doing home?' I asked him.

He shrugged again, an annoying habit he was getting into, along with his depressed moods.

'What's that supposed to mean?' I asked, exasperated.

'Nothing,' he said, his voice beginning to rise. 'Just that – nothing, *rien du tout*, nada, zip. I can't find a decent job this side of the Milky Way.'

I rolled my eyes heavenward. His definition of decent and mine were miles apart. We'd discussed it a million times. He wanted and felt he deserved the instant $40,000-a-year job. I felt that something much more modest with potential for advancement was far more realistic, but we didn't see eye to eye on this one. He didn't know that my own salary at the library was a great deal less than $40,000.

'Oh for God's sakes, Mum. You expect me to wash dishes at minimum wage.'

'I didn't say that and I don't want that anymore than you do, David, but expecting to make a lot right way is unrealistic. You have to be prepared to start lower and move up. That's how it's done.'

'Not anymore it isn't, Mum. Where have you been? There's no job loyalty out there anymore. Employers lap you up, that is, if you're lucky enough, chew you over and then spit you out when the flavour doesn't suit them anymore. That's what they just did with me. There *aren't* any more forty- and fifty-year careers with the same company. And even guys working that long aren't safe any more. You remember Joey? His dad worked for forty years and they let him go two years before retirement. Now they don't have to pay him a pension. How am I supposed to compete in a climate like that? And how am I supposed to accept eighteen grand a year when my last job paid thirty? It's demoralizing.'

What was I supposed to say to that? He was right – you couldn't take your job for granted anymore. I copped out and changed the subject, and soon wished I hadn't.

'How's Joey doing? Has he got over his divorce? Still living at home?'

'Yeah,' David said, scrunching up the chip bag and jamming it in the wastebasket. 'Why would he ever want to leave? He has it all. A nice room, home-cooked meals, laundry done for him, no rent payments ...'

I gaped at him: we could have been talking about David himself. But he didn't seem to notice the look on my face, and he continued –

' And he earns twenty-five thousand a year. He told me last year that he's saving all his money hoping to maybe put a down payment on a little bungalow. How can he do that now when he's just forked out all his savings to buy a second-hand Harley Davidson?'

'I don't know,' I said uneasily. David didn't say anything. In the silence, I tried to sort out my thoughts: here was a friend of David's with a good-paying job who chose to remain at home. I had assumed that once David got a good job, he'd move out – after all, that's what Bryan and I had done. But what if he didn't? What was I supposed to do to help him get back on his feet? I looked at him sprawled on the couch and suddenly felt so guilty. Bryan's words of the night before echoed in my head: 'Maybe we've failed him somehow and that's why he hasn't been able to make it out there in the real world.' Why couldn't he make it on his own, I asked myself? Why hadn't things turned out the way we had expected them to? Where had we gone wrong? Or had we?

* * *

Rebecca and Bryan need to review their relationship with David. They have lost the image they had of him as a successful adult, and this has made them feel they have failed him in some way. They need to understand why he has come home and why their guilt is misplaced.

Why Are They Coming Home?

Bryan and Rebecca are typical of all those baby boomers and their parents who were raised in a world where the sequence of events was laid out for all to follow. You grew up, went to university, got a job, settled down, married, had children, and created a home of your own. Nothing in that scenario hinted at returning home again. Young adults were simply not supposed to return home. For all parents, the goal was to lead their children to independence as soon as possible.

Loss of Good-Paying Jobs

The goal is still the same – to teach one's children to live independent lives – but it isn't as easy to reach as it used to be. Rebecca and

Bryan, growing up in the 1950s and 1960s, never had to worry about finding a job: they knew that with the right education the jobs were there for the taking. You could expect to work for a single company for your entire working life. Loyalty between employee and employer was taken for granted: you did your job well, and you were rewarded. Jobs are now much harder to find, and good jobs with good growth potential and interesting opportunities are snapped up in an instant. The competition for such jobs is intense, and it seems that no matter how well you perform you could wake up one day with no job as a result of enforced downsizing, bankruptcy, obsolescence, or redundancy (1).

David did everything he could to position himself for the job market, but his job was made redundant, and now he stands in the job search line behind all the baby boomers. The unemployment rate for those, like David, between 15 to 24 is much higher than for any other age group – and it doesn't include all those who have given up looking (2).

Jobs Don't Pay What They Used to Pay: Economic Fallout

All across the board, the younger generations have lost ground: wages are declining, and so is the earning power of their dollars. Today's young adults are earning less now than their counterparts in the 1970s. Entry-level salaries simply have not kept pace with inflation. Past generations could always expect their children to do better than they did; today's parents are witnessing a fall in their children's living standards, and can no longer assume that their lives will be better economically. This is reflected in the number of young adults returning home or never leaving in the first place. Yet assumptions die hard. No parent wants to accept that their child may end up with less while working just as hard.

Many young adults return home because their salaries simply cannot support their high monthly rent. It's a dismal prospect – working all day for a paycheque that just allows you to make ends meet. Many of these 'boomerangers,' as they have been called, miss the lifestyle they enjoyed while living with their parents. They see their old home with new eyes, and find it impossible to achieve a similar lifestyle on their own. Many are willing to give up their independence to live at home. Those who do so are hoping to save money to buy their own home, or to earn enough to be able to afford to marry, or simply to have some disposable income for a car or a stereo.

Staying Home to Survive the Financial Crunch

Many young adults are returning home for economic reasons; many others are delaying leaving in the first place, often because of the poor economic climate and poor job prospects. Many are delaying marriage and staying home to save money for the future. Many are staying in school longer, in search of the knowledge that will make them indispensable to an employer. Young adults entering, or about to enter, the job market today have seen the writing on the wall and realize that to compete with everyone else, they must be well educated.

Rather than living in a cockroach-infested apartment with an unreliable roommate who throws nonstop parties or never pays the rent, they have chosen to return home or stay home to save money while they learn. Many families simply cannot afford to support a young adult who has chosen to attend college or university while living away from home. Rent for an apartment is too much and so they attend classes from home.

Other Reasons for Returning Home

Many students come home because they find they need the self-discipline imposed by their parents to get their homework done and avoid failing. They find that living in residence or in an apartment with friends is not conducive to good marks. So they return to the place where they learned self-restraint, where parents make the rules and demand that homework be done.

But it's not just job losses and careers as students that bring young adults home, or keep them there. In an age when divorce has become all too common, the failure of a relationship can send them racing for home. In times of hardship and crisis, they come home with emotional needs that can be met nowhere else. Relationships are not the only catalyst here: *any* emotional crisis, whether it results from the death of a loved one, or an accident, or mental illness, or depression, or drug and alcohol abuse, can bring children home to regroup and reassemble themselves in an environment where they are loved and wanted.

Why Do Parents Feel So Guilty?

The return of a young adult can spark many feelings, not the least of which is guilt. Many parents convince themselves that somehow, in some fundamental way, they have failed to provide their children with the tools for making it on their own. The dreams and expectations they had for their children have come tumbling down, and they blame themselves.

This can be very stressful. Parents, like Bryan and Rebecca, who see their child's return as failure on their part and feel guilty about it should realize that in the vast majority of cases the learning of independence is an ongoing process, that a return is not a failure but simply a need to regroup before moving – a necessary, temporary crutch.

Guilt can be paralysing. It can blind you to what you must do *now*, by making you think only of past mistakes or *perceived* mistakes. Looking back at your past, and picking out things you might or might not have done as evidence that you have failed your children, is counterproductive. One single mother allowed her adult son to move in with her in a tiny one-bedroom apartment. His father refused to pay any more money, and his mother felt so guilty about the divorce and the horror she had put her son through that she let him sleep at all hours, demand the car, and generally walk all over her. Her guilt let this continue and prevented her from looking at the situation objectively.

Another mother gave her adult daughter free rein when she returned home because years before, when the girl was twelve, she had given permission for the daughter to have an operation to save her life. Unfortunately, the operation also left her sterile. From that day forward, the mother blamed herself for all her daughter's problems, and the daughter capitalized on this, and even reinforced her mother's guilt through her own belief that her mother owed her something for her 'error.'

We have had it branded into our minds that when our children hit eighteen they become, instantaneously, full-fledged adults. When they don't live up to the billing on the dotted line of time, no wonder guilt tends to creep in. Yet we are all different. Little Mike didn't walk until he was eighteen months, yet Josie walked at eight months; Dan talked at nine months, but Steve didn't utter a word until he was three years old. We all mature at different rates, physically and intellectually. Some children mature quickly, or have goals they can achieve only after they have left their parents. Some leave home very early; others leave much later, having taken longer to reach the point where they feel confident enough to want to leave home. Many leave and return several times before finding their own lives independent of their parents. It's a long, hard road to independence, and nowhere does it say that every young adult must travel exactly the same road on exactly the same schedule, generation after generation. We are setting our children up for a fall when we don't take into account that the world changes constantly.

Today's parents must realize that in earlier generations it was much easier to leave, and not just because of economics. In the 1950s sex before marriage was taboo, divorce was rare, there was no birth-control pill, and children were expected to be seen but not heard. Adults had priority, and the rules in place were rigid and made most adolescents want to leave home as soon as possible – meaning, as soon as they could get a job and support themselves or (in the case of many women) as soon as they could marry.

Returning home was not much of an option because the generation gap was far too wide. Children raised in the sexual revolution no longer considered it a sin to live together unmarried, and could not go home again to parents who would never understand those values. But the gap today is far narrower, and children are closer than ever before to their parents, and this makes living at home when the going gets rough a much more popular alternative than in the past.

For most, the return is temporary. But if there is no driving reason to leave – if they have it all and there is no need for independence – then it can be difficult for parents to get them to leave.

One father set his daughter up in a 'granny' flat and gave her credit cards and access to the family car. She had no need to leave, and without any responsibilities she did not mature to the point where she *wanted* to leave, until she got bored. Adult children who come home and have all their needs taken care of may be quite happy to give up their independence for security and financial well-being.

How Do Your Children Feel about Returning Home?

When an adult child returns home, parents should use their return to develop a new relationship. Consider this: If you feel guilty at their perceived failure, what must *they* think? Try to put yourself in their shoes. What are *they* feeling? *Why* are they home?

Returning home is not easy. Many boomerang children feel they have failed, and envy their friends who have made it. It was exciting and stimulating living away from home, and it is often discouraging to move back. They have become used to living on their own and to doing things their own way; now, suddenly, they have to swallow their independence. They may be wondering if they will ever be able to leave home and make a life for themselves. They may be depressed and unsure of themselves.

Moving home can be a real blow to any adult's pride, self-esteem, and self-confidence, and the worries of what the future holds can seem overwhelming. Most do not return home by choice, no matter what the precipitating event, and the return is usually temporary. Unfortunately, many people see young adults who return home as moochers and cop-outs scurrying home at the first sign of trouble. This is unfair: in any age group there are some deadbeats, but most boomerang children are home to regroup before leaving again.

Suggestions for Coping

Give them space. Don't nag them about finding a job, patching up a relationship, or doing better at their studies, as Rebecca has been doing. It applies unwanted pressure. Instead, be interested, supportive, and encouraging. You don't want to cause guilt trips by harping on a subject too often. Support them, and be a friend, but also remember you are a parent no more. You must let them solve their own problems, unless they are too ill or depressed to do so, at which point you will need to consult your family doctor. You must resist the urge to move in and take over. You must learn to draw the line between comforting and overprotection. You must also learn how to live with each other again in an evolving relationship that is based on mutual respect. Read on!

* * *

I'd had a horrible day at work. Someone had insisted we had a reference book on an obscure herbal remedy, and when I did a search and exhausted all avenues he insisted I was incompetent and made a loud scene. Then some kid's cat got into the library and caused havoc before we caught it. It took an hour to reshelve the books it had knocked down in its panic to get away from us.

I scooted out of work just ahead of rush hour thinking of the blessed half-hour of peace I would have before having to go out and buy groceries for Mum. She didn't sound or look sick anymore, but she said she still felt too wobbly to go shopping.

I pulled into our driveway and slammed on the brakes. The rusted wreck of one of David's friend's cars was taking up both spots in the driveway, and there was no room for me or for our neighbour's car. I cursed under my breath and backed out and parked on the street, hoping I wouldn't get a ticket. As I walked past the strange car, I glanced inside. The sight of make-up and a drycleaned frilly pink blouse draped over the back seat made me uneasy. Had David, who was supposed to be pounding the pavement for a job, brought a girlfriend home? I wasn't sure how I felt about that.

My head was throbbing as I pushed the key in the front door and opened it. I was nearly bowled over by the music blaring from the radio. I clenched my teeth as I strode to the offending box and switched it off. Unfortunately, the music continued as a dull pounding rising from the basement, where David had been sleeping ever since Peter balked at sharing a room again. David had been furious about being relegated to our mostly unfinished basement while his kid brother got a whole room to himself. He'd even tried to oust Danielle from her room, suggesting she might like the tiny, makeshift basement bedroom David had fixed up for himself. That'd be the day. We'd had some nasty rows over who was entitled to what, but the house simply wasn't big enough for everyone to have what they wanted. We still hadn't resolved it, and tempers were pretty thin. I stared at the radio and wondered why on earth David had felt he needed two radios going at the same time. He hadn't even noticed that one had been turned off, for God's sake.

I yelled down the stairs, fooling myself into believing David would actually hear me, and considered whether to go down and see what was going on. I actually got halfway down the stairs, carefully stepping over his discarded shoes and a heap of magazines, my anger simmering at the mess I saw. Then I heard a woman's voice during a break in the music and my courage fled. I rushed back upstairs, unnerved, upset, and not knowing what to do.

I hightailed it to the kitchen to make a cup of coffee, but the sight of the dirty dishes piled in the sink I had left spotlessly clean that morning made me want to cry. But crying wasn't going to help. David had never done the dishes before, so how was I supposed to change that? Furious, I washed the dishes. Then, with the music still throbbing through the house, I stomped into the living room, which was directly over David's space, making a lot of noise to let him know I was home. Then I slumped down in a chair and tried to read a magazine.

What were they doing down there? He was an adult but he was also my son. Was he entitled to do whatever he wanted in my house? How could I tell him to entertain his female guests somewhere else? What was I supposed to do?

Tired as I was, all I wanted to do was curl up and snooze on the sofa, but I couldn't even do that. David's visitor's coat was draped on the sofa, and I knew she wouldn't leave without it. I wanted my privacy but I didn't want to be forced to go hide in my bedroom in my own home. I also didn't want to meet David's friend in the frame of mind I was in, so I went out and sat on the back deck and read my magazine.

I waited until I heard the music stop and David's friend leave by the front door, and then I followed him back downstairs and confronted him. He was sprawled across his futon as I barged into his room. He jumped.

'Jesus, Mum, you scared the hell out of me. I didn't know you were home.'

I was so taken aback by what he looked like that I lost my train of thought. He had shaved his head bald except for the tiny black dots that marked the abrupt end of every one of his silky locks.

Before I could stop myself I blurted out, 'God, David, your head looks like a bowling ball. Why on earth did you shave it all off? Who the hell is going to hire you with a head like that? You don't have lice, do you?'

David just stared at me and said nothing at all. I suppose I should have known better and stopped, but I was on a roll now. 'And while we're talking about looks, I really think you need to lose some weight, David. Those pants were huge on you when you arrived home and now they look like a skin transplant. It's all those chips and pop.' I waved my hand at the empty bags overflowing his wastebasket.

'I'm not a kid anymore, Mum,' he said quietly. 'You can't tell me what to eat or wear. If I want to eat chips and drink pop and get fat and wear tight clothes, that's my business now, not yours.'

I stared at him open-mouthed while he sat in the middle of the tornado he called his room. I couldn't see any *room* in it anywhere: a week's worth of laundry on the floor, his makeshift brick-and-plywood desk piled with dirty dishes and chip bags, books everywhere. I wondered what on earth he meant about not being a kid anymore. He hadn't even learned how to take care of his own laundry, and here he was talking about being an adult? But then I asked myself, with some misgiving, whose fault was that? I'd never given him the chance to do the laundry. Well, not really true. It had always been easier to just do it instead of constantly nagging him about doing it. But that had been when I knew it wouldn't be forever. Now that it did look like forever, I

didn't think it was such a great idea at all. But I didn't know what
to do about it.

David looked at me and sighed. 'Mum, would you say this sort of
stuff to your best friend?'

I frowned, trying to pick up the threads of our conversation.

'You know, Mum, tell her her hair looked awful, that she was fat
and her clothes looked rotten?'

Now it was my turn to sigh. 'Would your best friend do your
laundry and cook your meals and clean up after you every day of
the year if you were perfectly capable of doing it yourself?'

Stalemate. We were eyeing each other like boxers in a ring when
we heard the front door crash open, followed by Bryan bellowing
David's name. We could hear him stomping down the basement
stairs.

When he stormed into the room he took one long, hard look at
David, showing no sign that he saw his shaved head, and exploded.

'I ran out of gas in the middle of rush hour! I learned swear
words I never knew existed from the drivers I held up!'

David said nothing.

'I missed an important business meeting,' Bryan went on, 'and
the excuse that my son forgot to fill up the car as he had promised
sounded pretty flimsy. What the hell is wrong with you? Just
because your Chevy bit the dust last week doesn't give you carte
blanche on my car.'

'It was almost empty when I took it out,' said David, throwing up
his hands. 'Why should *I* have to fill it up? I put a couple of bucks
in to bring it up to where it was. I can't afford any more. I'm unemployed, remember? Besides, it's not *my* fault you ran out of gas. You
should have looked at the fuel gauge.'

Oh boy, I thought, looking from father to son – now we're in for
it. Bryan was struggling to keep a semblance of sanity and searching for the right words when the doorbell rang. We all stared at
each other for what seemed like forever. Then David leapt off his
bed and ran past us, calling over his shoulder –

'That's Joey. Gotta go. I'll see you later. I'll eat with him.'

I yelled after David: 'Where are you going? When will you be
back?'

'Mum, I'm not a kid anymore. I have my own life. I'll be back when I'm back.' And he disappeared, followed more slowly by a seething Bryan.

Why did I think we were operating under a double-standard here? Why did I think that telling someone where they were going had nothing to do with being a kid or an adult but everything to do with common human courtesy? Where had we gone wrong?

Bryan's anger was still simmering when I found him in the kitchen nursing a coffee.

'Who the hell does he think he is?' he asked in a strangled hiss. 'He comes running back home to Mum and Dad when his job is declared redundant, complains about where he has to sleep, borrows the car and leaves the tank empty, eats a huge amount of food without helping to pay for it and never wants to tell us where he's going. Who the hell does he think he is?'

'He's our son,' I said quietly.

Bryan looked at me as though I'd failed kindergarten.

'Of course he's our son, but he's walking all over us. It was fine when he was a kid, but now he's an adult and he expects us to treat him like one in all the convenient aspects, but let him be a little kid when it comes to money, car ...'

His voice trailed off and I finished his sentence for him.

'... laundry, dishes, vacuuming, grocery shopping, responsibility.'

'What about us, Rebecca? What about the good times we were going to have when the kids grew up and left home? You realize that if Danielle and Peter follow in David's footsteps we'll be old and sick by the time we're together again, just you and me.'

'It's not all bad, Bryan.'

'I know, I know, he's fun to have around most of the time. But it's not what we expected for ourselves, is it?'

We looked at each other and wondered what the hell we were supposed to do to regain the harmony of our lives. Do we kick David out? Do we let him stay and make some rules? Do we coddle him? Do we badger him?

* * *

Many parents complain about their boomerang children. But at the same time, recent research indicates that most get considerable enjoyment out of having their young adult children living at home – as long as it's temporary. They also appreciate the extra help that many of these boomerangers provide in terms of household chores and social obligations (3, 4, 5, 6, 7). Most adult children who choose to return home enjoy fairly comfortable relationships with their parents. That much is logical: adult children who *don't* get along with their parents, who are unwanted and unloved, are less likely to come back. Yet even in the best of relationships, neither side enjoys the petty irritants that can pile up and cause big problems if they aren't dealt with early.

Reverting to Old Roles

When a young adult moves back home, suddenly the family is faced with uncertainty and ambiguity. There are new demands and new expectations. How they are handled is critical to the smooth running of a household.

Initially, the easiest route is simply to fall back into the old, familiar parent/child roles, which is what most of us do. If you always cleaned up after your children and made their meals and disciplined them and laid down a curfew, you simply take up where you left off, even if your child is now in his twenties. But resentment can build up on both sides. The child is a 'child' no longer, and picking up after him or paying his bills begins to pall on the parents. At the same time, the parents are 'parents' no longer; the young adult does not want to be treated as a child, and finds it frustrating to be ordered about and given a curfew. Yet he may still perceive his parents as parents and not as individuals in their own right; consequently, he may fall back into the old role of dependent son. Mum and Dad always did these things for me when I lived here before, so it seems natural for them to continue now that I'm an adult.

Except that things change. Like many adults who return home, David expected to find everything the same. In the meantime, however, his two younger siblings had matured, his half of the bedroom had been taken over by his brother, and his mother had gone back to work. When young adults come home for a short visit they often don't see any changes, because parents often try to make things appear as they have always been, cooking meals, doing laundry, and following all the old routines. After all, they know their child is just there for a visit, and they want to make it a good visit. Even siblings fall into the old routines for a short time. But when the visit lengthens to an indefinite stay, no one can expect to keep up the charade for long.

One stay-at-home mother who waited on her husband and son for years found a job and a new life once her son left home. When he returned, she reverted to the old ways, looking after both men as she had in earlier years. It was too much. She had been able to do it for her husband and still hold her job, but she wasn't able to do it for two grown men. Because of her new job and other interests, the old demands on her time were no longer welcome on a permanent basis. She rebelled, and father and son began chipping in and helping at chores they had never helped with before.

Evolving Relationships

Parents and adult children have their separate lives to live, and the young adult who comes home must take on responsibilities she perhaps never had to take on as a child. She has to realize that the home of her childhood is no longer the same. Nothing remains static: the players have all grown older. The children are now adults with adult values and opinions. If the generations are to live together in harmony, the old parent/child relationship must evolve into a new adult/adult relationship. In these changed circumstances, it's critical for each side to understand how the other is reacting and feeling. Boomerangers must be able to see their parents as human beings with wants and needs, and parents must see their boomerang children as adults. Only then can they become friends.

The Power of Respect and the Taking On of Responsibilities

Parents and adult children must learn to treat one another with respect and demand it in return. They have to learn to operate on a level of peers, as friends, not as a parent and child. David is right when he asks his Mum if she would criticize her best friend, and Rebecca is right when she asks David if he would expect his friends to do his laundry and cook his meals. They're close to seeing each other's side. Now they must work to communicate what they feel and resolve it, as friends would.

How easy is it to shift to the role of a friend when your children return home? The answer depends a great deal on how you raised them and on the relationship you had with them when they were young. If you gave them plenty of independence early on, showed them respect, and expected them to take responsibility for more things as they grew older, then the transition will not be as difficult as if you did everything for your children and never encouraged them to help out around the house or solve their own problems. If you were strict and controlled every aspect of your children's lives, it will of course be more difficult for you to begin to treat them as adults – but that is precisely what you will need to do.

Many parents begin to develop a solid relationship with their adult children only after they start setting limits and treating them as adults with responsibilities that must be met. One of the more painful things you have to do as a parent is force yourself to stand by and watch your children struggle to solve a problem. Moving in and taking over does not teach children anything, except that they can always lean on someone else when the least little thing goes wrong.

As your children grow older, your authority and control must involve mutual respect; otherwise you will find it difficult to move into an adult/adult relationship. Be mature. Be willing to share, and be willing to admit when you are wrong. Many parents are afraid of losing face in front of their children. But a refusal to admit you are wrong only leads to resentment building up in your child. They know you are wrong and don't know why you won't admit it. They learn from you. Parents must realize that they need to show they are not perfect – that they are human beings with goals and problems, mistakes and fears. By admitting mistakes, you are showing your children or adult children that they can make mistakes too and be forgiven. Respect is a two-way street.

Adult children who return home must take responsibility for

themselves within the family home before they can expect to do so outside it. They must be given responsibilities and follow through on them. If you are afraid they won't love you anymore if you don't do everything for them, then you don't have much faith in the ties that bind. It's not laundry and food that matters more here – it's love, and caring enough to gently make your children take responsibility for their lives. You're doing them no favours by waiting on them. You can be damned sure their friends, landlords, peers, and bosses won't wait on them or do their laundry. What boss ever did laundry for you?

Rebecca and Bryan erred when they allowed David to come home as their son and not as their adult son. They rallied around him in time of need but then didn't spell out what the new relationship was going to be. They need to lay down foundations in concert with David and his siblings so that everyone knows where everyone stands and what is expected. This should not be a one-sided process; rather, it should be done in an atmosphere of compromise, consideration, and respect.

Paying Rent or Doing Chores in Lieu of Rent

Money is a touchy issue with most families. People prefer to talk about almost anything else. However, if a young adult returns home and is making a good salary, parents should consider charging room and board. Many parents balk at this; in fact, many are adamantly against it – and so are their children. All feel it is insulting. Many parents feel that since they never had to pay their families board, they can't expect their own children to pay. After all, the room is still there and the rent was free before the child left home. It's still their home too, so why should they pay? It's unnatural to ask for rent, especially if the parents are not in financial need; however, for some families charging rent is a financial necessity and the child and parent have no choice. It seems that when there is a choice, most young adults do not pay rent. Several studies have shown that only about 25 per cent do so (5, 6, 8, 9).

On the other hand, if the adult child is able to contribute financially, asking for a token rent will give her a sense of responsibility and control over her life. By helping out the family, she will become used to honouring commitments and reaping satisfaction from doing so. If she is trying to save for a house and is doing so diligently, then it may be better to expect chores in lieu of rent; but if she is frittering away her savings, charging her some rent may help her learn how to run her financial affairs properly. There is no free lunch in the real world, and learning that at home is less painful than learning it out there.

The rent charged is usually a token amount, unless it is critical to the financial health of the family. It should be set through discussions between parents and children. Charging rent to an adult child who has no money and no job is, of course, ludicrous. However, rent does not have to be paid in money – indeed, even when the children can afford to pay money, many families find it easier to follow a barter system. Perhaps the son or daughter will be expected to fix something, or paint the porch, or do household chores (e.g., grocery shopping, cleaning, and meal preparation).

The young adult must take on some responsibility and contribute in some fashion to the running of the household. Daily chores, of course, must be shared by all. It helps to look at the situation in terms of a bunch of adults sharing a house. All are expected to do their share of the cleaning, cooking, grocery shopping, meal preparation, and other typical chores. As soon as the young adult is able to contribute financially, she should do it either formally, through a monthly rent, or informally, through buying food and gas for everyone at regular intervals.

It is helpful if the young adult knows what it would cost to live in comparable fashion somewhere else. One set of parents had a daughter who balked at paying $150 per month; they changed her mind by taking her apartment hunting so that she could see the going rates. Some parents feel that charging rent to a young adult who can afford it is important, but they put that rent money, without telling her, into a trust for her to use once she is back on her own feet. Studies have shown that parents who charge rent or ask for chores in return for housing are more likely to be successful in their relationships with their adult children (5, 6, 8).

Guidelines

Everyone in the household should help establish household guidelines. (Don't call them rules! It's like waving a red flag if you do.) A new deal must be worked out that reflects the changing lifestyles of both parents and their adult children. When a young adult moves back home, clear adult expectations must be set down. Of course, if you have always treated your child as an adult there will be much less trouble with this, as mutual respect and consideration will have been well established already. Schedules for various duties and chores should be set up so that all those involved know where they stand.

Rebecca is seething over the dirty dishes in the sink, the loss of privacy, the dirty laundry, the messy bedroom, the loud music, and David's friends coming over unannounced. Instead of talking it over with David in a rational manner and bringing her feelings into the open, she sits on them so that her resentment builds up. Bryan is no better: he expected David to put in more gas than he used, but didn't tell him as much. David replaced what he used, and didn't understand why his father was upset.

You cannot expect others to read your mind. Believe it or not, if you don't tell them how angry something makes you, they may never learn. So tell them frankly but nicely, and then use that to begin a dialogue to find out what bugs them.

Set down guidelines for who does the dishes and when, who buys the groceries, who makes the meals, who does the laundry, and who helps get groceries for Grandma and Grandpa. The simplest approach is to make a list of all the chores and have people underline the ones they want to do and the ones they don't. Then pool the lists and divide up the chores accordingly.

Privacy Issues

When your newly minted adult returns home after a sojourn living away, the house can suddenly seem very small and transparent. Both for parents and for adult children, one of the hardest things to get used to is the lack of privacy. Common space must be used in consideration of others. Private space should be treated with respect. Knock before going into another person's bedroom – even a young child's, and even if the door is open. It is a simple signal of respect to do so. Mutual respect reinforces rather than loosens a relationship. Lack of respect breeds resentment and distrust. If you treat your children as adults, they will begin to respond in kind; if you treat them as children, they will rebel. No adult likes to be treated as a child. Giving a curfew to an adult is begging for trouble and shows a lack of trust and respect. Of course, if the adult child is abusing that trust by coming home drunk and noisy at 4 a.m. you will need to lay down the law.

Set down other guidelines for the common spaces – the bathroom, TV room, kitchen, and living room – and also for the TV and telephone. Talk over these issues in an atmosphere of mutual respect. Put yourself in your son's shoes and ask if what you are demanding is reasonable. Don't ground him from using the phone if he is always tying up the line. If it is a huge problem, suggest that he get his own line or, if that's too expensive, suggest that he make the bulk of his calls during certain hours so that he doesn't tie up the line indefinitely. Ask him to pay his own long-distance costs.

Before talking things over with your adult child, make sure that you and your spouse have come to mutual conclusions about what you both want. You have a right to your own home, and you have a right to impose certain rules, but you need to work together as a couple and present a united front.

However, you must be prepared to be flexible. If every time your daughter turns up the radio you shout at her to turn it off, tension will slowly build. She must be free to listen to a reasonable amount of music. Things can be scheduled so that you are in the kitchen, or outside, or basking in the white noise of an air-conditioned bedroom while the music's on. A two-dollar set of earplugs, used on occasion, has defused many a fight over noise. Earphones have done the same. After all, you can't deny something reasonable to your children, and if you show them flexibility they will likely show you some in return. Patience and understanding go a long way to making life livable for all.

A Question of Values

On issues such as smoking, sex, religion, and politics, compromise may be impossible. If it is, you must have final say in your home. Your adult children are, after all, just guests.

You must stick to your own lifestyle and expect your adult children to respect it while they are living under your roof. If you don't smoke and they do and it bothers you, don't let them continue – you can be sure a landlord would not. If they are born again and begin preaching to you and you find that offensive, take them aside and tell them you respect their freedom to believe what they believe and they must respect yours. Avoid dressing them down in public: if they have done something wrong, tell them so in private, so that you leave their dignity intact.

Adult children develop values of their own that are not necessarily those of their parents. Sex, like money, is often a difficult issue. Parents who have no qualms about their adult children sleeping with their lovers outside the home often balk at allowing them to share a bed under their own roof. If you are uncomfortable with your adult children sleeping with unmarried partners under your roof, say so. Make the issue one of values. As long as your adult children are in your home they must respect your values, even if they do not agree with them. It is the price they should be willing to pay as mature, considerate adults for the comforts of home. The same applies to the use of drugs and alcohol.

It is a sign of disrespect if your adult children refuse to abide by your values while they are guests. If they cannot respect your values in your own house, you may have to tell them to leave. Your adult children have no right to impose their values on you unless the tables are reversed and you are living with them in *their* home. Unfortunately, there are times when parents and their adult children do not have the flexibility or sensitivity to resolve issues. Counselling (see appendix for resources) may be necessary; if that fails, the family may simply not be able to live together.

Remember that living with anyone involves compromises and obligations. Abusive or nagging behaviour is no solution to anything; building mutual respect *is*. Tension will be greatly reduced if everyone understands that the return home is temporary. If you and your children can develop a relationship of mutual respect on an adult/adult footing, it will be much easier to move into the next phase of the sandwich, when your children must help their grandparents face old age.

For more information and/or resources on ideas touched on in this chapter, see the appendix on resources.

CHAPTER THREE

The Second Slice of the Sandwich

The phone rang just as I was leaving for work, and I had to race back in to get it before whoever it was disconnected.

'Oh, Rebecca, I'm so glad I got you before you left for work.' My mother's voice was a whisper. 'Would you mind picking up a heavy parcel at the post office for us?'

'Mum, can it wait? I promised David I'd meet him after work and go over his job résumé with him. He's got some interviews coming up and I offered to help. Is it that heavy?'

'Not after work, Rebecca. I was hoping you could swing by and pick me up over your lunch hour, in case it's too heavy for me.'

'Mum, I can't. I have a lunch meeting. Why can't you do it yourself? If it's too heavy, leave it and we'll get it tomorrow.'

There was a long pause at the end of the line.

'Mum?'

'I'd hoped you could also drive me to my optometrist's appointment.'

Alarm bells went off in my head. She'd never asked me before to drive her to her appointments. I'd picked up groceries and little things like that since Dad had broken his hip – nothing much, really – but never had she asked to be driven somewhere. She was very independent and loved her little car and loved to drive. She'd taken over most of Dad's care and had had no trouble managing most things after the first few weeks before Dad could walk again. Her eyes were OK, so it couldn't be that. The only other thing I could think of was her car.

'What's wrong with your car, Mum?'

She hesitated, 'Nothing, really, but I have to park so far away and I'm still fighting this wretched cold so I didn't want to walk. But it's OK, Rebecca. I can do it myself somehow.'

Boy, could she ever make me feel guilty, but there was nothing I could do.

'You could always splurge and call a taxi this once, Mum, if you don't think you can park close enough.'

There was a long silence at the other end, and then she said –

'Could you at least drop off that book for me after work?'

How could she have forgotten already that I had to help David after work? I felt a spasm of fear. Was she losing her memory?

'All right, Mum, I'll try.'

The following day, Saturday, I was washing the windows – the ones Bryan had promised to do for a year – when I saw the bus pull up near our house. I stood and watched in surprise as my mother slowly made her way off the bus. A passenger offered to help her but she waved him away impatiently. As she walked down the sidewalk toward our house, I was aware of a slight hesitation in her gait, as if she was afraid she might fall. I'd never noticed it before, and my heart sank: suddenly she seemed old and vulnerable. How could this be the same woman who had raised four children and cross-country skied and played tennis – albeit with less and less vigour, until she was seventy-eight? In two years she had aged rapidly and had given up playing tennis and skiing. I wondered how much caring for Dad had taken its toll.

I ran down and opened the door for her.

'Where's your car, Mum? Why did you take the bus?' There was no danger here of a long walk. She had always parked on the street and walked the ten feet to our front door.

She ignored my questions as she moved into the living room and selected a chair.

'Rebecca, you said you'd drop off that book for me yesterday but you never came.'

'Sorry, Mum. I got tied up with David.'

'But you said you'd come, Rebecca, and you know I needed that book very badly. I can't sleep so well at night, what with your father's needs and all, and books help me get through.'

'You could have nipped over yourself – you always have before. I told you I had to help David and that I'd *try*, Mum.'

'No you didn't,' she said doubtfully and then quickly changed the subject.

'Speaking of David, his hair looks terrible. You should suggest he buy a wig. And get one for Peter, too.'

When Peter had seen David's hair he'd gone and borrowed his brother's razor and shaved his own, too. I could have killed them both.

'It'll grow back, Mum,' I said, trying to sound civil.

She looked so tired, and I felt a pang of guilt sweep through me. 'Where's your car, Mum?'

There was a long silence. She started to say something three times, and each time the silence fell again. I became alarmed.

'What is it, Mum? Are you OK?'

'I'm just fine, dear, if they could only find a cure for old age.' She cleared her throat again. 'It's just that I don't have a car anymore that I can use.'

Visions of a nasty fender bender flashed through my mind and I blurted out –

'Were you in an accident? Are you hurt?'

She looked at me, her face a study of confusion and hurt and something else I couldn't identify.

'No, not exactly an accident.'

'What is it then, Mum?'

'They won't let me drive anymore, Becky.'

She never called me Becky unless she was really upset.

'I failed my driver's test,' she said. 'They say I can't see so well anymore and my reflexes are too slow. What do they expect of an eighty-year-old with arthritis anyway? But I thought maybe the doctor would sign something to say I have to be able to drive. Your father can't anymore and we'd be lost without the car.'

I felt like a heel. No wonder she'd been irritable and demanding in the last few days. She had been scheduled to take the exam four days before – I'd even coached her on the metric system for the umpteenth time. But then I'd forgotten to ask how it went. What were they going to do without a car? Dad, when he'd turned eighty, had refused to take the driving test and had simply given up driving. It occurred to me that they would use me more, and I felt guilty for feeling the burden of that even before it had begun.

'I'm sure the doctor can do that for you, Mum.'

She stared at me.

'I mean, sign something for you, to say you can drive.'

'Have you forgotten that I went to see him yesterday by bus, Rebecca?'

I *had* forgotten! She'd taken the bus because I couldn't drive her there.

She stared at me in ominous silence and then said, 'He refused. Said in all good conscience he couldn't allow me to drive anymore even if I did retake the test and pass.'

I was embarrassed and didn't know what to say. Why hadn't she told me about her licence yesterday? Maybe I could have found a way to drive her. I wanted to help but didn't know how, so instead I awkwardly patted her hand and then scooted out to get some tea. When I returned I saw her struggling to take the lid off a jar of candies.

I walked over, set down the tea tray, and tried to take the jar from her.

'I can do it *myself* Rebecca,' she said, and turned her body away from me to hide her arthritic hands.

I was hurt that she had rebuffed me, and I didn't know what to say.

Suddenly in frustration she thrust the unopened jar into my hands. 'I can't do it. I can't even open a jar of candies anymore.'

*   *   *

Moving from Independence to Dependence

Rebecca is just starting out in her role as souciaire for her parents. As the years pass, a shift takes place in the balance of independence and dependence between the souciaire and the elder. The only certainty is that this shift will be different for everyone. For many souciaires it begins slowly; for others, it is precipitous, and follows an injury or stroke or other illness that disables the parent. For still others there may be no shift at all: the parents, blessed with good health, live independent lives until the day they die.

The fact that their parents are aging often comes as a shock to children, as it did to Rebecca. Although her mother at eighty is still fit enough to take care of her husband, the signs are that this may not always be so. Sometimes it takes a long time for children to realize their parents are slipping. Like Rebecca, they don't want to admit it. Watching your parents grow old and frail and vulnerable and in need of help is never easy. Studies have shown that most parents give to their children more than they receive in gifts, financial help, babysitting of grandchildren, socializing, counselling, and knowledge and advice. This seldom changes before the parents reach the age of eighty-five (1). Only when age begins to take its toll do parents begin to need more help than they give; at that point their children, instead of leaning on them, must let their parents begin to do the leaning. But it isn't easy. Because they've always seemed invincible, we often don't notice our parents slipping until we see the trash piled up outside the house, or dishes no longer cleaned, or the house messy and dirty.

Elder care is not restricted to any one age group. Some souciaires have elders who became disabled in their sixties; others have elders who functioned well into their eighties or nineties (by which time the souciaires themselves were old). Some will never have to care for their elders.

Because we are living longer and healthier lives than ever before, we have had to redefine the boundaries of old age. We have been pushing those boundaries back year after year to the point where more and more 75-year-olds – an age once considered very old – are active, independent citizens living full and healthy lives. Indeed, statistics show that the majority of our elders (70 to 75 per cent) live independent lives until well into their eighties, and remain at home until they can no longer cope. Sixty per cent of those over 65 and 40 per cent over 85 have no real functional limitations. More than 80 percent of those over 65 described their health as pretty good or very good (2). The perception that old age and ill health are synonymous is no longer true, except for those who are very old indeed.

The Help That Souciaires Provide to Their Elders

As they age, elders may require more and more help from family members in order to remain in their own home. Most elders want to stay in their own home and retain as much independence as possible, and this is where their families can be of help to them (2, 3, 4).

At first, elders may need only occasional help, from picking up the odd groceries or doing yardwork to dealing with tradespeople (mechanics, plumbers, electricians, and so on). More and more varied help may eventually be required, such as providing transportation, banking and financial help and advice, doing shopping, laundry, and housecleaning, and preparing meals. In many cases this type of help evolves into more direct personal care such as helping elders bathe, dress, eat, and take medication.

It has been estimated that 25 per cent of people over 65 need some form of assistance, with the amount needed depending on their state of health (2). Statistics Canada estimates that in 1985, 21 per cent of people over 55 needed some help with heavy housework, 12 per cent with groceries, 33 per cent with yard work, 7 per cent with cooking, 4 per cent with money management, 3 per cent with light housekeeping, and 2 per cent with personal care (5). The need for help increases with age. Thus, 22 per cent of 65- to 74-year-olds need help with heavy housework, and 12 per cent with groceries, while 46 per cent of those over 75 need help with heavy housework, and 33 per cent with groceries (6).

The amount of time souciaires spend caring for elders varies according to the needs of the elders. Souciaires tend to see their elders at least once a week and in many cases every day (7, 8, 9). One Canadian study showed that souciaires phone their mothers almost daily, visit three times a week (10), and provide a great deal of emotional help along with physical chores such as cleaning, transportation, and house maintenance (11). Those elderly who are still relatively autonomous may need only a half an hour or so of help a day; those who are more dependent may need three or more hours a day in order to remain in their own home.

When elders can no longer drive, their needs grow. Elderly people who lose the ability to drive lose far more than just a car. Rebecca's mother is quite typical in being angry and frightened about losing her licence. A large part of her independence has been wrenched from her; she is being forced to rely more on her daughter, and both of them feel helpless to do anything about it. Elders who can no longer drive have to face the fact that everyday chores such as shopping and banking are no longer as easy as they were. Such chores can begin to look insurmountable. Many seniors can no longer simply walk to the grocery store and carry or cart back groceries, and taking a taxi to the store is too expensive, and often too inconvenient, to be a workable alternative. Anything that restricts elders' movements may also restrict their independence and make them apprehensive about leaving home at all.

Some of the support that children give to their elders is not needed on a daily basis; in this category are emergencies, temporary illnesses, and dealings with institutions. When an old-age security cheque goes missing, it is often the souciaire who makes the phone calls to track it down. If the hospital needs certain forms to be brought in, or the bank says there's been an error in a statement, it is often the souciaire who takes over the responsibility. Indeed, souciaires often spend more and more time mediating for their elders with various institutions and helping them weave their way though the maze of health services that often faces them. Souciaires also give a vast amount of emotional support that is underestimated in terms of the time and effort behind that support. Such things as phone calls, outings, socializing, and sympathizing cannot be quantified easily and so tend to go unrecognized in the research literature. Yet according to recent research, women provide more emotional support than any other category of help (11, 12, 13).

That most of the assistance comes from family members (75 to 90 per cent of care of the elderly comes from family) (13, 14), dispels the myth that we don't care for our elderly the way our ancestors once did, and that most elderly live in institutions. In fact, only 7 per cent of our elderly live in institutions, and the majority of those who do are very old and frail. The most likely source of the myth was professional caregivers, who saw institutionalized parents almost exclusively and who did not see the countless souciaires in countless towns who were helping their parents remain at home for as long as possible, or bringing them into their own homes (2, 14).

One study showed that 78 to 90 per cent of elderly parents see their children at least once a week and are in contact with them roughly as often. About 80 per cent of elderly people have living children (15). According to another study, more than 80 per cent of aging parents lived less than a half-hour away from their children and about 30 per cent lived with their children – a drop from 60 per cent in 1960, to 33 per cent in 1980 (16). Most elderly people want to be cared for by their children if the time comes and not by strangers or social workers, although many have no choice in the matter because they either have no children or live far away from them, or are estranged (17).

*   *   *

'Mum! Mum!'

The tone of David's voice had me dropping the clean laundry all over the basement floor and hurling myself up the stairs two at a time.

'It's Grandma – she's feeling dizzy, Mum.'

He looked at me, his face blanched with worry.

I grabbed the phone from him.

'Mum? Mum, what's wrong?'

'I don't feel so well, Rebecca.'

'Where's Dad?'

'I had to ask a neighbour to take him to rehab and he's not back yet.'

I felt guilty. He had asked me to drive him and I couldn't do it.

'Maybe it's the pills,' Mum said.

'*What* pills, Mum?'

'They make the print on the bottles so small now, Rebecca – maybe I mixed up my medication.'

'I'll be right there,' I said in alarm.

I hung up and rifled my purse for the car keys. David came up quietly behind me.

'You want me to come?'

I could have hugged him.

When we got there, Mum was sitting on her favourite faded blue sofa surrounded by a batch of photos. She looked small and vulnerable and old, and I felt my heart lurch. I headed straight for the pill bottles beside her on the table.

'It's OK, Rebecca,' she said. 'I got out my magnifying glass and I haven't poisoned myself. It was a false alarm. I feel fine now. Sorry.'

I was relieved and so was David. As I put the pill bottles back, David reached over and picked up one of the photos.

'Who's this, Grandma?'

He held up a picture of my mother when she was forty years old, her long, sleek black hair flowing around her lovely face. Mum and I looked at each other, both realizing with a shock that David had never known his grandmother as anything but old. The look on his face said it all: he could see no resemblance between the forty-year-old in the picture and his grey-haired grandmother on the sofa.

'It's me David, when I was forty,' Mum said.

David stumbled for the right words, and to save him more embarrassment I hurriedly said –

'Have you eaten, Mum? If you haven't, it may be why you felt so dizzy.'

She shook her head as she began gathering up the old photos. Her hands were shaking as if she was cold.

'Mum, you have to eat,' I said.

I asked David to go and get her a sandwich and some juice. As he disappeared into the kitchen I found a blanket and folded it around her.

She shoved the blanket away.

'I'm not an invalid *yet*, Rebecca. I don't need your pity. I can still take care of myself even if I can't drive your father to rehab.'

She glared at me, but then her anger suddenly deflated and she looked away, embarrassed.

'Mum? What's wrong?'

I waited for what seemed like forever. When finally she spoke, it was in a barely perceptible whisper.

'I'm scared, Rebecca. Do you know what that means? I'm afraid of growing old. I can't even read the writing on my prescription bottles. I don't remember things very well anymore. I have to leave myself notes or I forget my appointments.'

'So do I, Mum. Everybody does.'

Her voice began to rise. 'Please don't patronize me, Rebecca. I'm not talking about a calendar or appointment book here. I'm talking about forgetting how many pills to take and when. I can't see as well anymore and the doctor agreed. I'm a hazard on the road. I have to turn the radio up high – when David comes in he always turns it down, so I know my hearing is going.'

'But it's natural, Mum, growing old.' What a platitude, but I couldn't think of anything else to say.

'Tell that to the billboard people and the advertisers. All those magazine ads and TV commercials make it seem as though the only acceptable humans on earth are under forty.'

'It's not that bad, Mum.' But even as I said so, I knew she was right, except that the cutoff was probably closer to twenty-five than forty. She looked up at me and took a deep breath.

'I'm afraid, Rebecca. I'm afraid for your father. What if I get sick and can't look after him anymore? I'm already having trouble. I can't drive him to rehab anymore, and he's missed some appointments because he hates having to ask for help and he can't handle the bus.'

I watched her hands toying with one of the photos. She looked up and caught my eye and smiled.

'I know you take him as often as you can, Becca. He can't find anything to do with himself, and I don't know what to do with him. What if he has to go into an institution and I can't go with him? What if we have to move out of our house and leave all our familiar things behind? I'm afraid of dying. I'm afraid it will hurt. What if I'm all alone? What if I die before your father?'

As she paused for breath, I sat down, too stunned to speak.

'What if he dies before me? How will we live without each other? Where will I go? I'm afraid I'll be alone. I'm afraid I'll die first. I'm scared I'll die last. I'm afraid of falling on a busy street, of not being able to carry my groceries. I'm sad I'll never see my grand-children grow up. I'm scared I'll die slowly and in pain. I'm afraid I'll go senile and be a burden on everyone. I have so much left to do. I don't understand where the time has gone. I have so many fears and doubts, Rebecca, and I can't talk about any of these things to anyone because it's just not the thing to do. You're not supposed to talk about death and growing old.'

She stopped and stared at me. I wondered how long she had kept these fears bottled up. I wanted to wave a magic wand and make it all go away, but I couldn't, and I felt lost. I couldn't make assurances that could never be true.

'You see? I've made you uncomfortable just talking about it.'

I sat there groping for words. She was right – I *was* uncomfort-able. It had never really occurred to me that she might be afraid, and I'd never bothered to find out what she was feeling. But if she was afraid, where did that leave me? If she couldn't look after Dad and herself, then I would have to step in and do it. I owed them that much. But maybe all she needed was something to do. Since Dad retired they'd been getting in each other's hair. Dad had made no plans, and his moping about the house was affecting Mum. Maybe if I got them involved in stuff, Mum would feel better about herself.

*   *   *

Growing Old: Losses Faced by the Elderly

No one wants to grow old and become infirm. We are the only spe-cies on earth that is aware of its own inevitable death, and that awareness can make old age frightening as bodily functions deteri-orate and cognitive abilities begin to wane. We know those things are the beginning of the end. How we handle them has much to do with how we view ourselves as people and how well we accept our own mortality.

Our elders must confront many losses and face many fears as they age, and souciaires must understand what these are in order to help them. Elders can develop many problems. Some develop them early in old age, some very late, and some not at all; much depends on their lifestyle and their genes. Often their energy levels fall and they are not as agile as they once were. They may not be able to form arguments as efficiently as in the past, and frustration over this can lead to irritability and a fear of things getting worse. Dementias in old age have been estimated to afflict only 15 per cent of the elderly; however, normal memory loss is not uncommon (18). Many old people greatly fear losing control of their world, and memory loss can affect an individual's functioning and self-confidence.

Physical losses such as those associated with arthritis, osteoporosis, emphysema, strokes, and heart disease place restrictions on seniors' movements, and they mourn their loss of independence. Any medications they must take can bring unpleasant side-effects; also, sleep disturbances, greater susceptibility to the cold, and poor nutrition are common among the elderly and can gnaw away at their self-confidence.

Knowing When to Help

Souciaires often find it difficult to provide the necessary care in a way that doesn't constitute interference or result in a loss of self-esteem. Rebecca's mother was angry with her daughter for trying to wrap her in a blanket. She was defensive, and saw Rebecca as treating her like a sick child and not as an adult. It frightened her to see herself becoming more dependent on her daughter, who was once totally dependent on her. Rebecca's mother needs some help, but she doesn't want it prematurely, and so Rebecca will have to evaluate the care she gives and make sure it is really needed and wanted. Elders are well aware of their losses and will be more sensitive to any care offered. Rebecca's mother saw in Rebecca's gesture a smattering of pity for an old woman. When children become more solicitous, it can be alarming for elderly parents, who still feel quite competent to handle most of their affairs. Their children may feel that their elders need help when in actual fact they don't. Be sensitive to how your parents respond to your help, and look for signs that the help is appreciated or needed. Many elders appreciate unsolicited help, so if you are unsure whether your help is wanted or not, ask first.

Elders Fear Being a Burden

Although most elders want and expect their children to help them, it can put them in conflict. They may feel they have failed to prepare properly for their future if they must be dependent on their children. They see things getting worse, and they know they need more help but feel they are a burden. Those who are still autonomous may worry that they won't know when the time has come to move into an apartment or seniors' facility. Even though they know they can't help needing help, it doesn't lessen their reluctance to accept it. Knowing they are a burden and that they are helpless to do anything about it may make them cranky. They feel guilty (as do their children). Rebecca's Mum lashed out at her daughter when she couldn't open a jar of candies. She was frustrated and angry and didn't want to admit she couldn't do it herself. There was another woman who refused to admit she could no longer knit. She spent many frustrating hours every day knitting and unravelling and knitting again in an attempt to finish a pair of socks she used to be able to do in a day. Souciaires must help their elders come to terms with their limitations by being patient and sensitive to both their needs and their losses.

Growing Old and Combatting Ageism

Seeing the outer manifestations of age in the mirror – the wrinkles and baggy necks, the drooping eyelids and hair loss – can be devastating. When old people look in the mirror they see *old*, but when they look in their minds they see *young*; this is because thoughts, in a functioning adult mind, are ageless. Yet every one of us can relate to David's feelings on seeing the photo of his grandmother. We have all seen our grandparents and marvelled at pictures of them when they were young. We find it hard to imagine them as ever having been young. Because we never saw them progress from young to old, we have no memories to flavour our current perceptions – they just look old. David cannot be blamed for not seeing in his grandmother the forty-year-old she once was. At the same time, most of us can remember our own parents when they were younger. When we look at them today we can still see the younger woman or man peering out from behind the wrinkles and the smiles. Souciaires need to remind themselves to look for that younger person every day, lest they begin to treat their parents as old in mind as well as old in body. This anonymous poem says it all:

A CRABBIT OLD WOMAN
What do you see, nurses, what do you see?
Are you thinking, when you look at me –
A crabbit old woman, not very wise,
Uncertain of habit, with far-away eyes,
Who dribbles her food and makes no reply
When you say in a loud voice – 'I do wish you'd try.'
Who seems not to notice the things that you do
And forever is losing a stocking or shoe.
Who unresisting or not, let you do as you will
With bathing and feeding, the long day to fill.
Is that what you're thinking? Is that what you see?
Then open your eyes, nurse, you're not looking at me.
I'll tell you who I am as I sit here so still;
As I rise at your bidding, as I eat at your will.
I'm a small child of ten with a father and mother,
Brothers and sister, who love one another,
A young girl of sixteen with wings on her feet,
Dreaming that soon now a lover she'll meet;
A bride soon at twenty – my heart gives a leap;
Remembering the vows that I promised to keep;
At twenty-five now I have young of my own
Who need me to build a secure happy home;
A woman of thirty, my young now grow fast,
Bound to each other with ties that should last;
At forty, my young sons have grown and are gone,
But my man's beside me to see I don't mourn;
At fifty once more babies play round my knee,

Again we know children, my loved one and me.
Dark days are upon me, my husband is dead,
I look at the future, I shudder with dread,
For my young are all rearing young of their own,
And I think of the years and the love that I've known.
I'm an old woman now and nature is cruel – 'Tis her
Jest to make old age look like a fool.
The body is crumbled, grace and vigour depart,
There is now a stone where I once had a heart,
But inside this old carcass a young girl still dwells,
And now and again my battered heart swells.
I remember the joys, I remember the pain
And I'm loving and living life over again.
I think of the years all too few – gone too fast,
And accept the stark fact that nothing can last –
So open your eyes, nurses, open and see
Not a crabbit old woman. Look closer – see ME.

Despite the ravages on her body, an eighty-year-arthritic old woman like Rebecca's mother may feel no different emotionally from the nineteen-year-old girl she once was. She has more wisdom and knowledge and experience, but essentially she is the same person caught in an older body. We are the product of our experiences – of what we have learned, of what we think and of what we do – no less at the end of our lives than at the beginning. Rebecca's mother is fundamentally still the same as she was sixty years ago. Most elderly are intelligent, alert, healthy, and involved; even so, they face an uphill battle in the PR department.

The stereotype of the befuddled old woman and senile old man is relentlessly reinforced by the media day in and day out either directly, through portrayals of elders as weak, senile, feeble, confused, forgetful, ugly, and frail, or indirectly, through the suggestion that life past sixty doesn't exist in this world of thin, nubile twenty-somethings. Rebecca's mother has a point. Advertising bombards the old every day, saying it is desirable to look as young and fit as possible. The saying goes that 'a person who ages well is a person who doesn't age.' If, as an elder, you still bear a startling resemblance to your forty-year-old past self, you are eulogized – you have defeated old age. If, like most of us, you actually look your age, then you have been defeated by old age. The media do the elderly and the rest of us no favours by preoccupying themselves with youth.

Elders can feel strongly that they have lost their usefulness to society. They fear becoming the stereotype that the ads make fun of, and this can lead to depression and sometimes suicide. After retirement they suffer a loss of prestige; they may feel as if their opinions are no longer sought and are therefore no longer valid or important. They fear losing the interest of others more than they fear death. Cumulative losses in physical and mental health can make elders housebound and inactive, and a spiralling dependency can develop. Depression is not easy to diagnose in the elderly, but if behaviour becomes erratic or exaggerated, souciaires should seek advice from their family doctor, if the parent refuses to do so (19).

Souciaires need to understand what their elders face. It is not always easy to empathize with elders, and often we react with impatience or ageist platitudes that marginalize elders even further. Rebecca's mother's ability to look back with satisfaction on her life will strongly affect how well she is able to cope with old age. If she has few regrets and views her live as having been meaningful, she will have an easier time facing the future than those who feel that time is running out and that they have not accomplished what they hoped. The inner strength that comes from accepting mortality, and the knowledge that one is free to do what one wants without all the social posturing of earlier years, can make old age a liberating stage of life.

How Well Have Your Elders Planned for Retirement?

The quality of elderly people's final years and the degree of care they will need from their children depends on their health and on how well they planned for their retirement, both financially and emotionally. Many elderly who live on fixed pensions worry incessantly about whether they will have enough money to see them through, while others refuse to spend a cent more than they need because they want their children to have it all – even if it means giving up some well-deserved rewards for themselves, such as travelling.

Those who make plans for an active life after retirement are far better off than those who wake up the day after retiring and find themselves with nothing to do. Rebecca's father did not plan for his retirement and now he and his wife have too much time on their hands and are getting in each other's hair. Rebecca needs to help them find a focus for their lives, which would help her mother stop dwelling on all her fears.

Those who plan well use their retirement to expand their lives and to explore new avenues in a way they could not when they were tied to a workday and a paycheque. For these people aging has many positive aspects. No longer do they have to worry about dependent children or the pressures of work. They can concentrate on their own needs and begin to do the things they always wanted to do but never had time to do. Elderly people who stay involved continue to feel needed and appreciated and good about themselves. This does much to dispel any fears they may be harbouring about their own mortality.

Suggestions for Keeping Busy

Try and help them to keep busy. Seniors have an enviable reputation as volunteers in just about every walk of life. They volunteer for an enormous range of activities and constitute a huge workforce.

Check out community resources, clubs, sporting events, children's libraries, hospitals, and museums. Help your aging parents find a new job or expand an old hobby, such as painting or stamp collecting, into something more. But at the same time, don't pressure them *too* much. Gather the information for them and present it to them, but let them decide. They must want to do it or it won't work; that being said, they may need the extra prod to get going, especially if they are unsure of themselves or fearful of change. Only you can be the judge of when prodding turns into excessive pressuring. (See the list of resources in the appendix for more information.)

But what if you can't communicate with your parents on an adult level? What if your relationship is stalled in the past and the more you try to help them the harder it is to satisfy them? What then?

*   *   *

My desk phone made a plaintive bleep as I was trying to finish work in time to beat the rush-hour traffic.

'Rebecca? We need some milk for dinner, and some other things as well.'

I sighed and said impatiently, 'OK, Mum.'

There was a slight pause, and then she added hesitantly –

'If you can't do it, it's OK, Rebecca. We can manage without.'

I took a deep breath and gritted my teeth. She'd caught me at a terrible time. I was late picking up David from an interview and in no mood for this and the spectre of rush-hour traffic too.

'I said it's OK, Mum. Read me the list and I'll be happy to pick it up for you. It'll be good to get a visit in too.'

An hour later I arrived with David and the groceries in tow. Both of us were in a terrible mood – David's interview had gone badly, and I suppose I hadn't helped matters by criticizing his choice of clothing. He hadn't actually looked that bad, with his hair growing back nicely, but I guess I had had to find some superficial excuse for someone rejecting my child. I rang the bell and then unlocked the door and kicked it open with my free foot. Dad was sitting in the living room listening to Beethoven, as usual, and Mum was reading a book. They looked as if they hadn't moved for weeks.

We put the groceries on the kitchen table. There were a couple of donuts on the counter and I eyed them hungrily, but with great resolve did not take one. It took us five minutes to stow away the groceries, and while we were doing that I called out to Mum in the living room –

'I filled out applications for you for a fitness centre that's just around the block so that you can get some exercise and meet some new people. You both need to get out more. They have a seniors' jazz dance class that meets every Tuesday and I've signed you up for that. I know how much you like jazz and the instructor says your arthritis will be no problem. They adjust the program for each individual's comfort level.'

When there was no response, I walked into the living room still holding some groceries.

'Did you hear me, Mum?'

She looked at me and sighed, 'Yes, I heard you.' But she didn't say thank you or anything, and that hurt. After all, they *did* need to get out. We'd been through it all a dozen times since Dad retired. He hadn't made any plans, and now the two of them were just vegetating. I couldn't let that go on.

Suddenly she pointed at what I was holding in my hand.

'You bought the wrong coffee, Rebecca. I said *ordinary* coffee, not that. Your father hates the decaffeinated kind. You know that.'

I stood there holding the coffee, suddenly feeling like a little girl who's just done something wrong. 'I thought the decaf would be better for you. Maybe let you sleep better.'

We looked at each other for a moment of silent sparring, and then Mum took the gloves off without even realizing it.

'I suppose you've already eaten the donuts so you'd better break out the cookies to go with our coffee.' She shook her head in resignation. '*Really*, Rebecca, why do you wear such ill-fitting clothes? I haven't seen your hips in years – they're always hidden under mounds of clothing. Instead of hiding your weight problem I don't know why you can't just lose it.'

I bristled at the criticism, and all the old feelings of resentment came surging toward the surface. How many times had she criticized my clothing, my weight, my hair over the years? My mother had never had a weight problem. She had never understood how hard I tried. And I *hadn't* eaten the donuts! She was just assuming I had. I stifled my resentment and went back into the kitchen to put away the rest of the groceries, just as Dad struggled in with his walker from the other door.

'I ordered a book, Rebecca, and I told the store you could pick it up tomorrow.'

I sighed to myself. He could have asked me first, but then he never had when I was a kid, so why would he bother now? He just assumed I'd pick up the stupid thing.

'By the way, Rebecca, we've got our income tax forms done but we'd like Bryan to look them over for us – you know, just to see if everything is all right and the government hasn't gypped us or anything.'

He was blustering, and I knew it cost him a lot to ask for any help at all. But I also knew he had no idea what effect it had on me. He'd never really trusted me with anything really important in all my life. Even though Bryan had no knowledge of finances and I had plenty, he couldn't bring himself to ask me – or worse, it hadn't even occurred to him to ask me. He saw me as his kid, and how can a kid offer dependable advice?

'I could do it, Dad.'

'That's a nice offer, Rebecca, but I think Bryan can handle it.'

As I ground my teeth at the way my father had dismissed my offer, David came in and got the pot of coffee and took it out to Grandma. Dad looked at me and said –

'A fine lad you have there. That was a really touching thing he did with his hair.'

'Touching?' It was not the word I would have used to describe David's meeting with the barber.

'Sure helped Joey, though, when he lost his hair. All his friends shaving off their own hair like that so he wouldn't feel so bad. David tells me the doctors are optimistic the treatments will work for Joey. But cancer's a scary thing – you never know. And it all happened so suddenly, too. Last week the world was his oyster, and this week?'

He shook his head sadly and hobbled out into the living room, leaving me grappling with the implications of our conversation.

I felt myself sinking into despair. You try so hard to do the right thing, and then *wham!* your kid turns you into an idiot, by doing something nice that you'd assumed was something exactly the opposite. Just the way my own mother had assumed that I would eat the donut, and the way Dad had assumed that Bryan would do better with the finances and that I would be happy to pick up the book. The bitter irony: I'd done to David what they had done to me.

*   *   *

Changing Roles and Evolving Relationships

Your relationship with your parents plays a large role in how you handle their aging and how you interact with them as you care for them. Caring for parents may reactivate old issues that have lain dormant for years, such as Rebecca's weight problem. Relationships vary widely in quality among families, but no one is perfect. Old problems rise again, and you must learn to deal with them.

The uncertainty and ambiguity of changing roles means it will be necessary to reassess and adjust, just as you have to do with your adult children. As you help your children less and less, you may have to help your parents more and more; the former will be moving toward independence and the latter toward dependence. This does not have to be a negative experience. Most children tend to enjoy the company of their parents as they do the company of their own children. There are few problem families in which relationships are poor and ongoing care is a nightmare. This is probably because parents and children who don't get along lose touch with each other, with the result that the elderly parents are later cared for by strangers. If your relationship with your parents has generally been a good one, caring for them will be much easier than if your relationship has been rocky. Some adults who never had their own dependency needs met as children have trouble meeting their aging parents' needs, especially if their parents were previously unloving.

According to one study, most children have little or no conflict with their elderly parents but both parents and children feel there would be increased conflict if they lived together (15, 20). The more contact parents and children have, the greater the potential for conflict in relationships, which are made up of many memories, both old and recent, pleasant and unpleasant.

Once you find yourself helping your parents more, unresolved or incompletely resolved conflicts over past deeds can rear their heads. These unresolved conflicts can affect the outcome of any current conflicts, which may or may not be related. Rebecca's resentment of past treatment of her weight problem does not allow her to shrug it off now; she remembers all the other times, and instead of confronting her parent with her feelings, or shrugging it off, she allows the resentment to build with each new incident.

The realization that your parents are vulnerable can soften past grievances. Understanding your parents and how they got to where they are today can also help you forgive and forget past hurts and see clearly what they need. Mary became a lawyer – and a good one – but her job became more difficult when she began having to care for her mother. Her mother constantly belittled her and criticized her career to the point that Mary thought her mother felt she was worthless. Actually, her mother was jealous: she had raised four kids and had had to give up her own legal career. By understanding her mother's jealousy, Mary will find it easier to ignore the criticisms as irrelevant; she will also find it easier to sympathize with her mother.

If in the past you and your mother or father have had tussles over parental control and authority, this is likely to continue. Your parents may have a hard time adjusting to the adult in you, just as you may have trouble adjusting to your own adult children. Rebecca may spend the rest of her father's life trying to prove to him that she is worthy of his trust. Even though she knows she is, she seems unable to get over her need for him to agree. Rebecca could have pointed out to her father that she was more qualified than Bryan to help him with his finances, but she didn't. She can bite her tongue and let it colour her relationship with her father; or she can bring the issue to a head; or she can just ignore it, reassess her role, and move into a new relationship. Mutual understanding is of course the best basis for relationships between parents and adult children, but if the parent (or child) has a permanent blind spot, the child (or parent) may have to learn to ignore it for the sake of harmony.

Parents Are Never Perfect

We often place our parents on pedestals, and look upon them as all powerful and unable to make mistakes. When we begin to find out they are not perfect it can be a blow. It is critical to realize that parents are never perfect and that we must allow them to be human. If they're not what you wished them to be, you must accept them as they are and forgive past conflicts. If you secretly resent that your dad never taught you to play football, or missed all your graduation ceremonies, or that your mother made you look after your kid brother, or refused to ever allow you to use her car, forgive and forget. If the transgression is unforgivable, as in the case of sex abuse, try at least to put it behind you. If you have always felt that your parents loved your siblings more than you, then either talk it out with your parents or let it go. Just don't dwell on it. If you are trying to help your parents, any anger and resentment from past relationship problems will colour your dealings with them and make caring for them difficult.

Mismatched Expectations and the Need for Communication

Conflict can arise if both sides have different expectations and don't communicate them. One daughter went to a lot of trouble every Thanksgiving to put on a big dinner for her parents and her extended family. She assumed that her parents, who had always hosted the dinner before they sold their home, would want the tradition to continue. In fact, her parents had grown to dread the yearly gathering because there were always too many people and the commotion was too much for them.

Communication is essential if you are to establish the expectations on both sides. One woman assumed that after the death of her father her mother would move in with her, and she made plans accordingly. When moving day came, to the daughter's great surprise the mother refused to go. People who know each other well, or think they do, are more apt to assume they know what that person wants. In fact they often do not.

This observation cuts both ways. Don't let your parents make assumptions either, and when they make incorrect ones, point them out politely. Rebecca should have told her father that she didn't want to pick up the book right away and that perhaps it could wait a day or two. By airing each other's false assumptions, a parent and an adult child can avoid many problems. Rebecca had assumed that her parents would want to join a fitness club. Her mother's lack of response raised a huge red flag that Rebecca missed. She interpreted the silence as ingratitude; in fact it meant, 'No, I don't want to do that.'

When children help their parents in areas where they don't want help, or fail to help them in areas where they do need help, both sides can become frustrated. A mismatch of expectations and needs can be avoided if parents and children communicate in a clear and honest manner that respects the feelings and needs of everyone involved. One mother went every Saturday to hear her daughter's choir, and confided to a friend that she really didn't want to go every week and would prefer a less structured arrangement. The daughter, it turns out, was making a big effort to arrange her mother's transportation in the belief that she lived for the event. Mismatched expectations had caught these two women in a rut neither of them particularly wanted.

Communication is a vital element in any smoothly running relationship. You must send clear messages, not ambiguous ones that leave the others involved wondering exactly where they stand. Most people beat around the bush when it comes to delicate subjects such as sex, death, and moving house. They don't want to hurt feelings or be seen as greedy or cold-hearted. A newly widowed father of four sons decided he wanted to sell the family home that had been in the family for sixty years. He asked his one son who lived in the same city if he and his wife would mind. Both gave him a variation of 'You know best, Dad,' which didn't help the father one iota. Meanwhile the son was harbouring a desire to move into the old home with his family. He didn't really want his father to sell; at the same time, his brothers, who lived in another city, didn't really care. In so many of our conversations we withhold an enormous amount of information, and this can cause damage. The father couldn't tell his son he wanted to sell only because maintaining the old home was getting to be too much for him. The son couldn't bring himself to tell his father he wanted to live in the old home.

Is There Role Reversal?

Some people perceive the role of children caring for their aging parents as a role reversal. According to Brody (2) the logic is that as the parent ages and loses mental or physical functioning, or both, he or she becomes like a child or infant. Role reversal it isn't. Lack of bladder control in an infant is incontinence in a parent. Infants struggle to gain, whereas the elderly struggle against loss. Old people are not cute like babies, and where a baby has milestones an elder has *millstones* that inevitably get bigger. Elders have a lifetime of experience, wisdom and memories, so when you help dress them or wipe their faces of food, it is not the same as doing so for an infant. Elders are *aware*, even if crippled by stroke or arthritis. Their bodies are betraying them so that they cannot take care of themselves, but if you treat them like children you risk damaging their self-esteem as well as your relationship with them. Society is preoccupied with youth, as is reflected in the media. Your aging parents have been devalued, so don't make things worse through thoughtlessness. You cannot become parents to your parents for the simple reason that while they took care of you at the beginning of your life, you are caring for them at the *end* of theirs, at a time when the outcome is inevitable. They need empowerment; they need to feel they are still in control. Try to make decisions *with* them, not *for* them. It is easy to project your own needs and wants on others, but often it is harmful. When you assume you know what elderly people want, you risk treating them like children and may be forcing them to give up their own opinions. If, on the other hand, your parent has many opinions and is highly critical and demanding of you, the two of you will have to sit down together and discuss how to resolve this. It is never easy to give up independence, just as it is never easy to become a parent's keeper. Both sides must allow the shift from independence to dependence to happen. Children must allow their parents to depend on them, and parents must allow their children to look after them.

You must be honest. The elderly are very quick to pick up on dishonesty, and feel unwanted and unnecessary when they are the targets of it. Saying in a cold, clipped voice, as Rebecca did, 'I'll be happy to bring the groceries, Mum,' is like throwing down the gauntlet. It was more than obvious by her tone that she was not happy at all to be doing it, and the added comment that she would be glad to have a visit was just pouring vinegar on the wound.

Power Struggles

Inevitably there is a struggle for power between souciaires and their elders. The elderly want to retain as much control as possible in as many facets of life as possible. If they are on a special diet and cannot stray from it, the souciaire must take control in a firm, polite way, but mustn't let this spill over into other areas, such as what clothes to wear, what brand of coffee to buy, and what to do in their leisure time. Elders often want care to be given according to their own preferences and may resist souciaires providing it differently. One souciaire bathed her mother's feet every day and always started with the right foot. But the old woman wanted her left foot done first, and they battled over it every day. There was no reason the souciaire couldn't have done the left foot first. It might have saved a daily argument and given the mother some sense of being in control, small as it was.

But sometimes the parent being cared for is too demanding or too controlling, to the point of tyranny, and souciaires often find it difficult to handle this. The psychological balance of power is often held by the parents because it has resided with them naturally for years. If your parents' demands are unrealistic, take a stand and explain why you feel the way you do. Talk it out and try to arrive at a compromise. If they still won't budge, you will just have to do what you feel is right and hope they will come around. You cannot let them bully you, just as they cannot let you bully them. Respect on both sides is important.

Learning from Your Elders

You are in the unique position of being a parent to your children and a child to your parents, and you will find many learning opportunities in both roles. In a moment of pure irony, Rebecca realized that in the assumptions she had made, she was doing to her son what her parents were doing to her. You ought to recognize that some of the problems your adult children face in dealing with you, and you with them, are mirrored in how you deal with your parents, and they with *you* – the adult kid.

You can continue to draw much support and emotional comfort from your parents. Take advantage of their wisdom and experience, and continue to seek their advice. They may feel their opinions are no longer important and be reluctant to help, but you should not stop trying. The evolving relationship can be stronger than it ever was as you and your parents accept your new roles and work together to achieve mutually satisfactory goals.

CHAPTER FOUR

Life in the Middle

The alarm clock went off much too early. Reluctantly, I hauled myself out of bed and did the rounds, waking everyone up before going downstairs to put on the kettle and get breakfast started.

As I was getting out the eggs, Peter came galloping into the kitchen, gulped down some juice, and said, 'Gotta go, Mum, last basketball practice before tomorrow's first round finals. You'll be there, won't you? And can you bring some pop?'

'What basketball finals?' I asked in exasperation. 'Peter, you never told me about any finals.'

'Oops, sorry, Mum. They start tomorrow, Friday, over lunch. Will you be there? I'll save you a seat.'

Before I could answer, David came in. Peter waved to me and disappeared out the back door.

'Tomorrow's my big day, Mum. First day on the job.'

I beamed at him as I beat the eggs in a bowl. It was a huge relief that he had landed an entry-level job at a nearby computer company as a software writer. I knew I had been anxious about him being unemployed, but I hadn't realized just how much until he came home with the good news.

'Can I borrow your car tomorrow to take my computer stuff to work?' he asked. 'It's too heavy to carry on the bus.'

I was about to answer when the phone at my elbow rang and David answered.

'It's Gramps,' he said.

I wiped my hands on a towel and took the phone from him.

'Hi, Dad, what's up?'

I listened in dismay as he told me that the company he'd worked for for thirty years had cancelled his pension. They were claiming bankruptcy, and he'd made an appointment for us to talk to them tomorrow to find out what was going on. He suggested that on our way back we should pick up Mum, or had I forgotten they'd been invited for dinner? I felt the old, familiar frustration of wanting to say no to his peremptory request but being unable to do so. In exasperation I heard myself say, 'I'll call you back, Dad, and we can plan it all.' I'd find some way. I always did.

Danielle bounded in as I hung up the phone and said –

'Mum, I forgot to tell you there's an information meeting with my counsellor tomorrow at five about the scholarship. It'd be nice if you could be there.'

Danielle had won a six-month full scholarship to study abroad starting after Christmas, and Bryan and I were really proud of her, but I wished she'd told me sooner!

I dumped the eggs into the frying pan, mentally trying to figure out how to do everything I had to do and still get to work. That's when Bryan came breezing into the kitchen tying his tie, and said –

'Don't forget lunch tomorrow.'

We'd arranged a special lunch together weeks ago, so that we could have time to ourselves. I'd already had to cancel it three times and couldn't bear the thought of cancelling a fourth time – Bryan had been so disappointed. But I wondered how on earth I was going to schedule all of this.

'We'll have to take your car,' he added. When I started to protest, he waved me down:

'Mine's got to go in for repairs tomorrow morning. It's falling apart. The brakes, remember? So I thought you could leave for work early, follow me down and give me a ride back before work, and then pick me up at lunch.'

I was saved from having to say anything by the phone ringing yet again. I whipped the eggs off the stove and went to answer. It was Ginette, my boss at the library.

'Rebecca, please don't forget about the meeting after work tomorrow. We're expecting all the staff to show up. And by the way, do you have last month's financial statement done yet? I need it to send copies to the board before the meeting next week.'

My heart sank. How was I supposed to juggle my time? I hadn't specifically agreed to do anything for anyone, and I felt a pang of guilt trying to figure out who to refuse. I loved my family, and wanted to be there for them. I also loved my job and hated to let anyone down. I was having to neglect Bryan and the kids more and more as my parents' needs grew larger, and my work was suffering and I knew that wasn't right. Still, I figured if I planned things just right I could drive David and Bryan to work early, and still get to work on time myself. Then I could leave a bit early at lunch to drop off the pop and see five minutes of Peter's game before picking up Bryan for lunch, make a quick appearance at the office meeting before going to Dad's meeting, drop him off, drive to Danielle's meeting, shop and then pick up Mum and Dad for dinner. It was doable – just. The problem was I just didn't want to do it. I felt helpless and guilty and frustrated that I couldn't give everyone what they wanted, including myself. I also felt angry, which immediately made me feel guilty again. Was I the only one who felt this way? As though I was caught in a revolving door and going nowhere forever? I felt tears pricking my eyes and fled to the bathroom before anyone could see me.

* * *

The Definition of Sandwich Generation

Rebecca is not the only one who feels overwhelmed by obligations to parents, family, and career. Several recent studies have shown that at any point in time the number of people caught in the sandwich is not enormous, and this has led some researchers to say the Sandwich Generations are a myth in the making (1, 2, 3, 4, 5). That being said, the chances over a lifetime of being in the sandwich are good and getting better as we live longer and delay having children. According to one study, the strict definition of members of the Sandwich Generation is this: average age fifty-one, with at least one dependent parent to care for and at least one adult child who has returned home (6). But the parameters of the Sandwich

Generation are far broader than this in the public psyche. The Sandwich Generations now include families raising young children at the same time as they are caring for their elders. They may not have an adult child who has returned home for the simple reason that none of their children is old enough yet to leave home, yet they are still torn between obligations to parents and those to their dependent toddlers and adolescents. Sandwiched families also include those whose adult children have never left home. Under this broader definition, an estimated 3.4 million Canadians currently are members of the Sandwich Generations (7).

Who Are the World's Souciaires?

Virtually all studies of the Sandwich Generation, and studies dealing with families caring for elders, agree on one thing: the vast majority of the world's caregivers are women. Less than 10 per cent of primary souciaires are men (8, 9). Thus, over their lifetime women like Rebecca find themselves caught up in the competing roles of mother, wife, worker, daughter, and daughter-in-law.

How Do Souciaires Feel about Their Role?

How does all this caring affect the Rebeccas of this world? How do they feel about caregiving? It is not unusual for souciaires to experience a wide range of emotions related to their caregiving. One day they may feel frustrated and angry at the disruption to their lives; the next day they may find joy and pleasure in the caregiving role. Frustration and anger are common emotions among souciaires. The presence of parents and adult children can make souciaires feel frustrated that their own dreams and goals are on hold. Rebecca had to cancel three lunch dates with her husband because of the needs of others, and is concerned that this will soon turn into an ongoing problem.

In order to find the time to meet everyone's needs, many women cut down on the 'easy' things such as entertaining and family time and time with their husbands. These things may be 'easy,' but few souciaires would give them up, given the choice. A souciaire often finds herself torn between not caring enough for her parents and shortchanging her family. Souciaires like Rebecca watch their husbands grow frustrated as their mutual plans are always being thwarted by others' needs. Husbands may see their wives' parents as demanding too much, and their own kids – particularly the adult kids – as doing the same. They may feel as if they are competing with everyone for their wife's attention. The free time the husband had been looking forward to spending with his wife has evaporated, and he wonders when their time as a couple will ever come. In the first Canadian study of the Sandwich Generations, researchers found that 50 per cent of the women in a sandwich situation felt it was hurting their marriage (10).

Those who spend a lot of time caring and who have made huge sacrifices, especially for the elderly, may resent such demands on their time and the resulting losses in social life and then feel guilty that they are not doing enough. Some souciaires feel that things will never get better until their elders die or the kids move out – and then they feel guilty about wishing that time would come.

Feelings of Guilt

Guilt crops up time and again when souciaires talk about caregiving: guilt about caring too little, about caring too much, about not quitting work to help family members, about quitting work and not bringing in any money, about putting children in daycare or not putting them in daycare, or about getting angry at their parents, or about getting impatient with their kids – or simply guilt that they are young and their parents are old. They want the best for those they love. When they can't provide it, rightly or wrongly they often feel like failures. Yet they often set themselves up to fail. The goal of many souciaires is to make those they care for happy. If they can't do that, they feel guilty. Yet they can't possibly guarantee that their children will find their dream jobs. And it may be unrealistic for them to expect to make their parents happy, especially if they are caring for the frail elderly who cannot be given back their mobility and independence – two things that would make them happy, but that a souciaire cannot supply.

Why is it that women feel such guilt? Guilt can be a powerful motivator and seems to play a role in nearly every aspect of women's caregiving. If their children have not reached their goals, they may feel they have failed to teach them all they needed to become successful adults. The rationale here is that their duty was to raise them from helpless infants, teach them right from wrong, and give them the groundwork to help them become happy and productive adults. Unfortunately, there are many points along the way where parents can make real or perceived mistakes. Then, if things don't turn out as everyone hoped, parents berate themselves endlessly. No one is perfect. People cannot go through life second-guessing themselves. As long as you did the best you could at the time, you must learn to accept the outcome. You must realize that you cannot be responsible for another person's happiness (9).

It has been suggested that when souciaires feel guilty about not making their parents happy, the guilt is the result of all the attention they received as children. They can never pay it back no matter what they do, and thus they feel guilty. Perhaps subconsciously, they feel that they must repay that debt, but they never can. The roles of child and parent can never be reversed: daughters can't go back and give their parents what their parents gave to them. This leads to guilt (9).

What do you owe your parents? What does Rebecca owe her parents, or does she owe them anything? Objectively, they chose to bring her into the world and care for her. Rebecca's choices in her situation are not as simple as the one her parents made. At the same time, the pull of love, duty, and guilt is strong, as is the biblical injunction to honour thy father and mother. Also, caring is a labour of love: most of us could never turn our backs on our parents and say we owe them nothing.

The parent/child relationship endures, even if the child does not like her parents, because it is a unique relationship. You cannot choose your parents or children the way you can choose your friends. Yet most families are mutually motivated to help each other. When they receive help from a family member they do not feel they owe a debt, the way they might with a friend. This mutual caring is part of what makes the family relationship unique – no debts are owed or owing, yet paradoxically, we owe each other everything.

Guilt has many facets and can drive you to do things you don't want to do or can't do. It is too easy to fear that you will fail to help your parents or children when they need you, or fail to make them happy. You may not be able to make your parents happy, or ensure a productive life for your children, no matter what you do. You must learn to accept that and not worry about it.

Feelings of Fear, Dread, Worry, and Frustration

Other feelings associated with being a souciaire to both parents and kids include fear and dread: Will I become an invalid like my parents? Will my children never have a life of their own? You look at your children and yearn to see them fulfil their potential; you look at your parents and wish you could find a cure for old age. Especially for a souciaire who is looking after elders the physical and emotional toll of caregiving can be very real. Marital problems, depression, anxiety, worry, and frustration are too common. Those who are caring for elders who are ill also experience feelings of helplessness, sleeplessness, low morale, and emotional exhaustion (9).

Many souciaires worry constantly about the needs of their parents and their ability to help. Some worry even if their parents need no help at all. These women fret about future needs that may never materialize. One businesswoman phoned her mother daily, checking to make sure she was all right. Her mother, though seventy-five, exercised regularly and was in excellent health. She finally bought an answering machine to keep her daughter's incessant worry from oppressing her. Another woman spent much of her spare time trying to persuade her parents to move next door to her in the country, because she was worried about how she would care for them when they needed her and wanted to set something up before that happened. This, even though her parents were fully autonomous and living happy, productive lives in the city, and likely to continue doing so for years to come.

Some elders demand a lot from their daughters, who often get very little recognition for what they do. Stories abound of daughters waiting hand and foot on their parents, running endless errands, cooking meals, and neglecting their own lives. Yet the parents barely notice. When the person receiving care does not acknowledge it – or, worse, criticizes it – the souciaire's stress levels can soar. She may feel at times that the younger and older layers are not aware of her own needs and do not understand the stress she is under.

Stress Levels of Souciaires

The amount of stress felt by souciaires depends on age and circumstances. The more autonomous the parents and children, the less the strain. The older the souciaire, the more the strain (because generally age and energy levels are related). Most stresses felt by souciaires come from providing care to the elderly, yet most women are not constantly overwhelmed by caregiving unless their parents or children are disabled and require daily and exhaustive care – a topic beyond the scope of this book. For most souciaires the caregiving is not continuous and the days filled with frustration, anger, and guilt are usually well outnumbered by positive times.

In a recent Canadian study of the Sandwich Generation, 77 per cent of women said they were coping well (11). Notwithstanding the occasional arguments and feuds over messy rooms and privacy, women enjoy the company of their children most of the time. Women find that their children are a source of moral support, and many say their children help around the house and help with caring for their grandparents. Most women also derive deep satisfaction from being able to help their parents – especially when the parents are openly appreciative.

Yet many women in the study were merely 'coping' or grappling with their situation the best they could (3 per cent said they weren't coping well, and 20 per cent said they were coping well only sometimes). This indicates that many women are vulnerable to the cumulative stresses of caregiving and may eventually reach a point where they can no longer cope, especially if the good days stop outnumbering the bad.

Suggestions for Coping

To avoid becoming emotionally and physically exhausted by care-giving, you must strike a reasonable balance. Being a souciaire does not have to be onerous, as long as you do only what you are able to do without compromising your own emotional and physical needs. Set priorities and make sure you include yourself in them.

Write out a list of all your needs and wants, the time needed for each one, and the priority it deserves in your life. Write out a separate list for every member of your family and for those for whom you provide care. Then compile the lists, being honest about which responsibilities should take priority. If the items from your own list have landed at the bottom of the ladder, then you are not being honest with yourself: some of your needs should be at the top. Do not let guilt be your master. You need to strike a healthy balance between altruism and selfishness.

If, for example, you cannot get away from your elderly mother even for a day, you need to develop a thick skin and not be quite so altruistic. This doesn't mean you have to become selfish – only that you need to ensure that your mother does not take up all of your time. It is not selfish to want time to yourself. Quite the opposite: personal time is part of a normal, healthy life, and if you ignore that fact you can become physically and emotionally ill. If in arranging time to yourself you must say no to a request, so be it.

Do what you are able to do without driving your own life into the ground, and don't feel guilty. If your parents expect you to visit once a week but you can only manage it once a month, be happy with that and don't feel guilty over something you can't change. If your kids expect you to make their meals, don't feel guilty about laying down the law and getting them to make their own. Like Rebecca, you must learn to distinguish between needs and wants. Rebecca does not need to drive David to work, or even attend Peter's last-minute basketball game, because they don't need these things: they *want* them but they don't *need* them. David can take a bus or taxi, and Peter should take responsibility for getting his own drinks. In such situations you must learn to ask this question: They want it, but do they really *need* it? If they don't, you must then ask yourself honestly, 'Is their want stronger than my need?'

In the best of all possible worlds you would be able to give all that is needed to those you love, and all would benefit – you would feel good, and they would feel good. But most of the time, compromise on both sides is necessary to prevent souciaire burnout. Give what you can without harming yourself; when you neglect yourself, you indirectly neglect those for whom you provide care.

Ask yourself if you are overdoing caregiving. Will things really fall apart if you stop helping as much, or if you get others to help more? Do your children really need to have you do their laundry? Will your parents really love you less?

Be honest with yourself. What is motivating you to provide care? Is it guilt? love? a need for approval? Don't let others lay a guilt trip on you. Caring for someone day in and day out, out of a sense of guilt or duty will impair your ability to balance your needs against theirs. It can also lead to resentment and more guilt.

You must learn to see your parents and children as they are, and not as you want them to be. Sympathize with failure and grin when they are happy, but do not blame or credit yourself or depend on other people's approval for your own self-esteem. You may never get the kind of approval you want from those you love, but don't let this dictate your actions. Some women feel they will never gain the approval of their parents no matter what they do. For them to keep trying in the face of this admission is a recipe for frustration, anger, and burnout.

Life cannot be lived always for others. You must save a little living for yourself. Make time for yourself and your family, and give yourself credit for all the work you do. Keep a sense of humour, and be positive. Above all, take time for yourself. Like Rebecca, you have problems and dreams of your own that are begging for attention ...

* * *

I looked in the bathroom mirror and stared at the teary-eyed face staring back at me and wondered where the time had gone. I suddenly felt sad and lonely. All I could see was a swarm of wrinkles playing havoc with my once-smooth face. When I looked sideways I could see the skin of my neck starting to droop. My breasts were sagging, and there was more of me than ever before despite all my attempts to exercise and diet.

Abruptly I turned my back. In anger at myself and the world, I bent down and picked up a wet towel someone had dropped and threw it at the wall. That's when I felt a sudden twinge in my back – I couldn't even get angry without something getting in my way. I remembered the joking laughter in my sister's voice the week before when I'd picked up a rake and complained of an ache –

'Getting old, are we?' she'd said, half in earnest.

Suddenly all my bones were aching and I was sure arthritis was lurking in every joint. Or was it just sympathy for my parents that was making me feel that way? I was beginning to feel all the niggly early-warning symptoms of my parents' full-blown ailments. I was facing my own mortality, and having looked at theirs, mine seemed lacking: I felt guilty even *thinking* about feeling old when the reality of their mortality was closer. But then I looked at my children, so full of energy and youth, and I felt sad. Where had the time gone? Would there ever be time for Bryan and me before we were too old to enjoy it? I felt too old to be a mother, too young to have to help my parents. With all the demands on my time, I couldn't figure out how I could do it all without doing less at work, and the thought of winding down my job left me stone cold. I couldn't help thinking about me, wondering about *me* and my goals and dreams and fears – important things that seemed to be getting lost in the shuffle. What about me?

*   *   *

The Needs of Souciaires

Indeed, what *about* Rebecca? What about her *own* life independent of all this caregiving? She does not live in a caregiving vacuum and must contend with her *own* needs and dreams, not just her feelings as a souciaire. She's at a stage in her life when she's ready to focus on herself, but as she cares for elders and children she is beginning to wonder if she will live through middle age before she has the freedom to do what she wants without having to worry about family. People like Rebecca often feel as if the empty nest will never come. She was finally ready to relax, contemplate retirement and travel, and forge a new, stronger relationship with her husband, when suddenly she was faced with new tasks. The unplanned presence of adult children and the need to help elders throw a spanner in the works. She has had to adapt and reorganize her life to accommodate first David and now her parents as they begin to need more and more help to remain autonomous. All this at a time when she is also having to deal with some important life events of her own, which are far from negligible.

Middle Age and Thoughts of Your Own Mortality

Like the average sandwiched person, Rebecca is a fifty-one-year-old woman. She looks in the mirror and realizes she is no longer young; she sees that the mortality now facing her parents square on is beginning to eye her from the sidelines with some interest. She is finding it hard to watch her parents age while at the same time wrestling with her own menopausal middle age and altered dreams. She is beginning to feel every twitch and is starting to think she's developing her parents' illnesses. She is struggling with the concept of her own mortality, while fearing theirs. The myth of old age as being frail and feeble can cause fear in the middle aged, especially those whose own parents are not in good health.

As everyone knows, middle age brings with it the first of the ailments that plague us as we grow older: weight gain, balding, beer bellies, hypertension, back, knee, and shoulder problems, and so on. All these things, once on the distant horizon, are now unwanted guests camped at the doorstep as a portent of things to come. Such changes can be stressful. Just thinking about them or fearing their consequences can increase stress.

Until middle age, most people never give their own mortality more than a passing thought – one day it will happen, but it is so far in the future that it doesn't really apply. As a child you were immortal and would never die, and if mortality ever raised its head you laughed in its face. But as you approach middle age you begin to realize that mortality isn't something that happens to others; it can and will happen to *you*. At middle age you are, by definition, at least halfway through your life and are beginning to feel some of the effects of aging. Rebecca, like all of us, must acknowledge in a healthy way her own mortality and learn to accept it and the wrinkles and aches and pains that come with it, and not dwell on it every time her back aches or her right toe hurts. She must accept herself as she is, and not try to be the billboard woman or the woman who has defied old age. Also, she must not neglect her own health needs or postpone them because of obligations to others or fear of what a doctor might say.

You may think about your own mortality more if you feel that you have not reached your potential, if you fear that time is slipping away and that you have nothing to show for your life – that the difference between what you hoped for and what you got is enormous. Witnessing your parents coming to terms with time running out is inevitable, but to realize suddenly that time is also waning for you can be a numbing revelation. You look back on all the other stages of your life and see clear milestones to gauge your progress: learning to walk, learning to drive, graduating, getting married, first house, first job, first baby, first promotion. As you age, such external gratifications are not as common or as easy to achieve, so you must rely on your internal reward system – your self-esteem – and accept where life has taken you. You must reassess the often grandiose goals of your youth and not mourn over failed hopes that in hindsight were unrealistic. If you set realistic goals for yourself in the first place – university degree, first job, first house, first raise – then, if you are honest with yourself, the gap between your goals and what you attained may be minuscule. If, however, your goal was to become a famous actor or a million-dollar singer or an NHL star, and if you never let go of that goal even though you know you had a better chance of winning the lottery, then you will feel time slipping away far more painfully than those who made realistic goals and by and large met them.

Mid-life Crises?

The middle years are often described as a series of crises, where marriages self-destruct, the children leave, depression is rampant, jobs change abruptly (or retirement looms), bodies wrinkle and fade, and life stutters from one body blow to another. Women have been bombarded by the media for years with all the negatives associated with middle age: the myth of the empty nest creating vast numbers of depressed women, and the myth of crazed females struggling through menopause. Middle-aged women have been told to prepare to mourn the loss of their fertility. They've been told that wrinkles and grey hair and sagging necks are ugly and need to be altered to keep them looking young, as if youth is the only prize worth seeking. They've been told that if they don't keep themselves looking young they'll be seen as middle-aged losers. They've been told they will likely live alone and be lonely at the end of their lives, and they know the little-old-lady myth is still rampant. They've been told to prepare themselves for the sudden vagaries of their husbands, who upon reaching middle age may suddenly quit their jobs to buy a boat and sail around the world, perhaps accompanied by an aerobics teacher half their age. Middle-aged men are defined in the media by their careers, their accomplishments, and their public life; middle-aged women tend to be defined by their biological and childbearing status (12, 13, 14).

For the most part, women have been fooled by the media, which are determined to make middle age sound absolutely horrific. Quite simply, it usually isn't. Rebecca, like most women, is unlikely to undergo huge changes at mid-life. Although the effects of menopause can be very unpleasant for many women, many other women have no psychological or physical symptoms, and few suffer from extreme or debilitating symptoms. Contrary to popular belief, most women do not mourn the loss of their ability to have children but rejoice in not having to deal with their periods any more. And contrary to the empty nest syndrome, most women do not spiral into depression when their children leave home. The small minority who do generally are those who stayed at home to raise their children and never worked or had outside interests, and never planned for the empty nest. This is not to suggest that mothers are not sad at the departure of their children, but rather that most realize their kids must go their own way, and quickly adapt to a life without them underfoot. The truth is that most women

caught in the Sandwich Generations – and Rebecca is no excep-
tion – actually look forward to the time when they and their husbands are on their own once again, and can rediscover themselves.
Of course, some may find it hard to find each other again, and may
fear it. After twenty-five years of sharing their lives with their children, they don't always find it easy to be thrown back together, with
no other responsibilities to interrupt them (12, 14).

Mid-life as the Prime of Life

Middle age should be seen not as a series of crises but as a time of
self-esteem and acceptance and looking at new opportunities. It is
a time for reflection – for evaluating your goals and dreams and
plotting a course for the second half of your life. Some people consider it the prime of life. It is a time when major decisions have
been made and are behind you, when mortgages have been paid
off and there is more economic freedom. You may have to change
your goals and alter your concept of mortality, but coupled with
this is the freedom to do what you want without the paralysing fear
of youth. It should be a positive time when you can expand and
grow. You may never fulfil your potential as you saw it in your youth
but that doesn't mean you can't fulfil it *now*, with the more mature
eye of middle age to guide your dreams.

Job Worries

Female souciaries who are coming to terms with their middle age
must also consider their work and how caregiving is affecting it.
Rebecca works full-time at the library, and like countless women
enjoys her job but is finding it more difficult to do while still caring
for her family and her parents. She worries about having to cut
down to part-time hours or even quit her job entirely in order to
provide care for her parents and have time for herself and her family. In her words, it leaves her 'stone cold.'
   She may also be worried about job security and early retirement.
If she retires at fifty-two to care for her parents, she will have some
twenty-five productive years left. She is unlikely to want to spend

them all unemployed, but society has not made it easy for her to care for her parents and children and work at a career at the same time. Although it is now considered acceptable for women to work, where do they find time to do all the rest that society still expects of them in terms of unpaid labour?

This is not an idle question. One Canadian survey (15) found that 50 per cent of employees provide some form of care to their elders. The majority of women today hold down jobs of all kinds, yet they are still expected to do most of the caring for children and elders ... all this at a time when the labour force of 45- to 54-year-olds is the fastest growing (having risen from 15.9 per cent in 1988 to a projected 21.8 per cent in 2000). Of women between 25 and 54, 73 per cent work; of women 55 to 64, 35 per cent work (16). In 1985, 28 per cent of employees over 30 were souciaires providing an average of 10.2 hours per week for parent care. Some of these hours must be taken from working time, as not all parent care can be accomplished after hours (17).

The Financial Costs of Caring

Women quite simply can't do it all. Because so many women work, there has been a decrease in unpaid working time available for care that is creating a crisis. The economics of families caring for their own creates a temptation for governments seeking to slash budgets. Hospitals are closing and patients are being discharged much earlier to their homes. Who will be there to care for them? Working women cannot help out during the day. Yet governments are pushing for more community care, which is a euphemism for unpaid care by daughters, wives, and mothers. Such care may work in favour of a government with an eye to the bottom line, because much of it is unpaid work. Yet the costs to souciaires, emotionally and financially in terms of lost days at work, often seem to be overlooked.

The financial costs to souciaires have a direct bearing on their lower wages and pensions and higher health costs. Taking time off to have kids, then care for them, interferes with career advancement. Many women resort to part-time work and forgo the possibil-

ity of landing meaningful promotions. An American survey
showed that 11 per cent of women had left work and 28 per cent
were considering it because of caregiving duties, even though most
of them did not want to do so (18). Another study showed that
women give up an average of 11.5 years out of the paid workforce
to be souciaires, compared to just 1.3 years for men (19).

And women who don't leave the workforce often choose less
demanding jobs for less pay. Women's average earnings drop
$3,000 the first year after having a baby and $5,000 to $6,000 annu-
ally for two further years (18). The wage gap is widest among 45 to
64 year olds; thus, when men are at the pinnacle of their earning
power, women are still struggling to catch up. Yet for more and
more women, work is as important as family to a sense of self (18).

To Quit or Not to Quit ...

A recent study carried out in Ontario found that working souciaires suffer guilt at not being able to help more, as well as anger at
getting no recognition. Sixty-two per cent did not change their
working life to accommodate their souciaire responsibilities; however, 20 per cent cut back their working hours and 16 per cent quit
work entirely. In the same study, 53 per cent of women still had
kids at home (20). When parents required more help, it was the
daughters rather than the sons who rearranged their schedules,
took time off work, or quit (9).

Those daughters who quit work to care for elders tend to be
under more strain than those who either don't quit or never
worked. Women who work and don't quit view their work as central to their lives – as a career, not just a job – and are better educated. Those who quit or are seriously thinking of quitting have
parents who are sicker and need more care. These women generally have poorer mental health than the working women. Many
who leave work to provide full-time caregiving do so because they
can not afford to buy care. Most who leave are sorry to go and miss
the interplay and stimulation, the status, the chance for promotion, and the money and personal development that went with
their jobs. These benefits derived from the feeling that what they

did was important. They feel they have given up something of value that was important for their self-esteem, and yet they still quit because they felt it was their duty to help their parents or children, or both. Rebecca has every reason to feel 'stone cold' when she contemplates winding down her job. She must think carefully and make very sure that she is taking her own needs into account, including the financial impact of the household giving up one salary. If two salaries are required to make ends meet, quitting work will cause financial hardship. On the other hand, many women who work at low-paying jobs find that they cannot afford to buy care for their elders and children and that quitting work to provide it themselves is their only alternative. Souciaires in low-income brackets therefore need financial assistance or subsidized caregiving by the government, or their employers, or both, if they are to retain their jobs while caring for their elders and children.

Some researchers have found that there are no differences between working daughters and nonworking daughters in the amount of caring they provide (21, 22). However, working daughters often share personal care and meal preparation, with paid professionals, and to a lesser degree with their husbands and other family members. During the working day, care cannot be provided by a working daughter, and that daughter cannot spend as much time worrying about caregiving. These women feel it is better to pay for care than to quit work or reorganize their work schedules. They are the lucky ones who can afford to pay for care. Other women must muddle along as best they can, and often their self-sacrifice is enormous. One woman who quit said that while she was working her mother could not demand 100 per cent of her time, but as soon as she quit her mother wanted 110 per cent (9).

Lobby Your Employers

Employers need to sit up and listen. Day care for children is a big issue on which many inroads have been made, but with elder care we are still in the Dark Ages. Dealing with parents is different from dealing with kids, and employers must learn to be flexible to allow for this. A refusal from a child to see the dentist at 3:30 p.m. is not as effective as a similar refusal from an eighty-year-old. You can pick up your child and carry her forcibly to see the dentist, but who among us could do that with our parents? Negotiations over caregiving can be time-consuming and difficult, and employers must show some flexibility so that their workers can take time off to drive parents to appointments, and take sick days when their parents are ill. The employees can quite likely make up the time. For many women the alternative – quit work – is no alternative at all. It often leaves them resentful and unhappy – and probably financially challenged as well, as the family's two incomes shrink to one.

Meanwhile, souciaires continue to struggle between what society expects of women and what women now expect and want for themselves. And they are beginning to ask themselves – quite rightly – just why it always seems to be women who do all the caregiving.

*   *   *

I actually managed to get through Friday relatively unscathed. I'd done as much as I could for everyone, and I was exhausted. I flopped down on the lawn chair beside my mother on our back deck for a quick break before helping with the dishes, and heaved a huge sigh.

'Did you get to Danielle's meeting?' she asked.

'Yup, and I managed to see part of Peter's game, but I missed seeing him score a three-pointer because of lunch with Bryan, then I worked almost until quitting time, showed up for five minutes at my meeting ...'

I paused, and there was an awkward silence before Mum finished my sentence for me –

'... and took your father to that silly meeting and then rushed to make Danielle's information meeting and bought groceries for dinner for all of us, then came back to pick us up for dinner. Today isn't all that unusual, is it?'

She stunned me with her insight into my situation. Considering how she had been behaving recently, I'd almost forgotten that most of the time we got along really quite well. I was surprised that she'd noticed how much I'd been doing for everyone day in and day out: there were weeks when I thought no one noticed. Then I felt guilty at her insight, thinking perhaps I'd made her feel as though she was a burden to me. She must have seen the surprise on my face, and then the guilt.

'Don't think I don't know what you do, Rebecca,' she said gently. 'I know, I know, I've been critical and snarky and demanding since your father broke his hip, but that doesn't mean I don't appreciate what you do for us all. I'm a woman, remember? I've been there too. I'm still there.'

'Been *where*, Mum?'

'Looking after kids, giving up a chance at a career, looking after your sister when she came back after the divorce, looking after your kids, and now looking after your father. It's a caregiving career, Rebecca, and few women don't get promoted to it.'

I stared at her and realized that while I had thought she didn't appreciate what I was doing for her, I had never really appreciated just what she had done for me and was now doing for Dad. The strain of it was etched on her face.

'What does being a woman have to do with it?' I asked.

'Do you see Bryan looking after me and your father, and doing all the housework?'

'Of course not. You're *my* parents, not his.'

'You think that matters, Rebecca? I looked after your father's parents for years before they died.'

I looked at her with some consternation and began to think of all my friends who were caring for their in-laws. And then I thought about Bryan's parents, who were thinking of moving closer to their son, and felt my heart begin to race. Was this a never-ending treadmill I was on?

'How did you do it all, Mum?' I asked, trying to keep my dismay to myself.

'I never had to look after my own kids and my parents at the same time. I also had you young and never worked at a paying job. Mind you, caring for all my family has been a lifelong career with its own stresses. I've had many days like yours.'

She laughed suddenly at some memory only she could see.

'But I've had good times too,' she added. 'Your sister was a great help to me when she moved back, and you've got David – he's been helping around the house, helping us too, and I know you enjoy having him back. I can see it in your face.'

'But I feel so guilty,' I said. 'I feel I'm short-changing you and Dad, my kids and Bryan. You were there for me when I needed you. I need to be there for you too. But I need to be there for my family as well.'

At that moment Peter came out onto the back deck.

'Gramps can't find the Beethoven,' he said, 'and Dad says we're out of cookies.'

I looked at my mother in resignation and reluctantly got up from my chair.

'Why is it always us?' I asked.

She shrugged her eyebrows in a knowing way that made me smile and said –

'Because we always say yes?'

* * *

Caregiving Careers

Rebecca's plaintive 'Why is it always us?' and her mother's knowing shrug will ring familiar bells among today's families, especially among women: it is not just a perception on Rebecca's part, but a fact, that women provide most of the caregiving to adults and children.

It has been estimated that women can expect to spend seventeen years looking after their children at home and eighteen years (up from nine in 1900) looking after elders at the same time or sequentially. Eighty-nine per cent of women will be souciaires of children, or parents, or both, at some time in their lives (18, 23). Those who claim that the Sandwich Generations are a myth in the making are doing women a disservice – caregiving is a societal constant.

Most women provide caregiving for most of their lives, from raising children to caring for their parents. When grandchildren arrive on the scene, grandmothers often provide taxi service to schools and provide babysitting and other services. When the time comes, it is usually the woman who cares for her aging husband because she is likely to outlive him. The odds are good that she will live alone at the end of her life with no built-in souciaire, because she will have outlived her husband.

Simply put, women live longer than men; and since men usually marry women younger than themselves, it is no surprise that women are far more likely to care for a dying spouse than the other way around. They outnumber men two-to-one over the age of eighty-five (24). Indeed, a woman has a one-in-four chance of outliving her own son. Women outnumber men four-to-one in caring for severely disabled parents, and even when sons are the primary souciaires, it is safe to assume that their wives contribute a great deal (9).

Since most elderly are female, the most common caregiving scenario involves daughters caring for their mothers. More than 50 per cent of women can expect to become souciaires to their parents, and this percentage is likely to rise as we live longer. And parent care is not a single, time-limited thing: it may have to be faced many times. Many souciaires also help another relative; some care for two or three, either at the same time or serially (9).

Why Is It Always Women?

Why is caregiving a women's issue? More and more women like Rebecca are asking this question as they juggle full-time work with family. Traditionally, it has always been women who have cared for their children and their elders; quite simply, it is viewed as a woman's role. In virtually all cultures the nurturing is overwhelmingly a woman's job. Centuries ago only the woman could care for an infant – what man can breastfeed his newborn child? Since she was confined to the home, the role of souciaire to the elderly, and housekeeper, and cook, naturally fell to her while the man went hunting. This served society efficiently over the centuries: women who did not work were simply expected to mind the home fires and care for the young and old. Times have changed, but expectations have not: working women are still expected to fill the roles that had been theirs when they did not work. In actual fact, in the recent past caregiving was a shared responsibility; many women had wet nurses and servants to help with the children, and elders did not live as long. Nowadays, however, caregiving seems to fall solely on the woman. It has been deeply ingrained in most women that it is a woman's responsibility to care for both elders and children. Women take the responsibility very seriously. They've grown up in a society geared to it, unfair though it may be (25).

Girls are educated early in the souciaire role, and boys in male roles, as they watch and copy their parents. Television continues to show little girls caring for dolls and playing the helpless bystander, and little boys bashing around with guns and baseballs. Movies show boys in dominant roles, girls in nurturing roles. Most women are so well trained in their roles that research has shown that they just assume that if their brother agrees to look after the parents it will actually be the daughter-in-law who provides all the care. Other research indicates that women feel *they* should be the ones to alter their working schedules to accommodate caregiving, rather than their brothers or husbands (9). The roles die hard.

Things are changing, but very slowly. The long-running comic strip *Hi & Lois* has Hi reading to his daughter about a prince rescuing a helpless princess from an evil dragon. Dot asks why the women in fairy tales are always so helpless. Hi, unthinking, replies, 'Because it makes the story more exciting.' His little daughter is not amused. The next panel has Hi ad-libbing the story and having the princess slay the dragon. We need far more of this to help young girls and boys see each other as human beings and not as stereotypes, which harm both sexes.

Getting Men More Involved

Roles are often self-perpetuating, but they don't have to be. In families in which there are role models of caring, nurturing men as well as women, the roles can be reconstructed so as to be spread more evenly to reflect the fact that most women now work. Teaching sons and daughters to be equally comfortable in the kitchen, cooking and cleaning up and caring for others, and in the backyard, playing baseball or other sports, is a necessary first step.

When both parents share all the chores and caregiving and partici-
pate with their children in sports and other activities so that no
chore or activity or caregiving task becomes labelled as male or
female, we'll be a lot closer to a society in which all members share
the caring.

Men and Women as Souciaires

All of the above doesn't mean it will be easy for women to share the
load, or for men to take it on. The female compulsion to care,
which has been drummed in from an early age, makes it hard for
most women to refuse to help when asked. Rebecca's mother
pointed this out when she said to her daughter, 'Because we always
say yes.' Women feel pressure to be souciaires. They also set very
high standards for themselves and then feel guilty, as Rebecca
does, when they can't achieve it all.

Most women want to help and do so willingly: they have seen
their mothers caring for children and the elderly and learn by
example that that will be their role too. Daughters develop a
mutual helping relationship with their parents that is lifelong.
Research shows that caring for elders does not occur without a history of aid prior to the parent becoming dependent on that aid.
For years before their parents need help, daughters offer it anyway.
They gradually increase the level of help when they see that their
parents need it (26).

Women tend to feel responsible not just for physical care but for
emotional care, for parents and children alike. Rebecca is typical.
She feels responsible for everyone's well-being and wants to please
them all but is beginning to realize that she can't do it all – that it
was a fantasy for her to think she could.

Research shows that women provide more emotional support to
their family than men. Married daughters feel closer to their parents than sons and maintain closer contact with their mothers than
sons do. Older men are less connected to family than older
women, who see their children more often, regardless of distance
(8, 9, 17, 27, 28).

Generally, sons are able to distance themselves better; they feel less guilt and find it easier to accept that they cannot make their parents happy. They rarely feel responsible for the emotional state of their elders, perhaps because their role models were not nurturing men who looked after them but rather men who went to work and expected a hot meal on the table when they returned. Women need to learn some of this objectivity from their male folk. They need to learn, as soon as they can, to spread the workload among their family members and stop feeling guilty over things they cannot control.

The Power of Myths Affecting Women's Caregiving

Women are handicapped by the pervasive myths that feed their compulsion to care. For years mothers were told that by putting their children into daycare they were depriving them of all manner of things. These working mothers were blamed for everything from an increase in child delinquency to bedwetting children. That there is no evidence for these allegations doesn't seem to matter: the myth is strong, and women still fight it every day. After their children are born, many successful career women go back to work for a year or two and then throw in the towel, unwilling to leave their children in daycare and endure the insinuating comments of friends and business acquaintances that they cannot be good mothers if their children are in daycare.

A related myth that compels women to superhuman efforts is the one that parent care is not as good as it was in the good old days. The myth continues that we don't take care of our parents the way our ancestors did, that the caring family does not exist anymore, and that most elders live isolated lives, shut out from their families or dumped in institutions (29, 9).

Hatched more than thirty years ago, this myth seemed to be supported as fact by the increasing numbers of elderly living in nursing homes in the 1970s and 1980s. Far from being an indication of abandonment, this merely reflected that more disabled elderly were living to be very old, to an age at which nursing care was likely to be necessary. Their numbers and disabilities made them highly visible, and the professional caregivers who looked after them maintained the myth – understandably, in that they saw mostly old people in institutions who either had no relatives, or were alienated from their families, or who were far too sick to be cared for by family. Meanwhile, the vast majority of elders were not being institutionalized but were living independent lives longer than ever before in their own homes and with help from their children (9). Researchers agree that most elderly have frequent contact with their families and are not isolated at all. The number living with their children has decreased over the years, but for the most part this simply reflects better health. The majority of elders see their children at least once a week, and most more often than that (9, 10, 30, 31).

Middle-aged women are actually doing more than their parents ever did to help adult children; they are also working and volunteering more and providing more emotional support to their elders. Souciaires make real sacrifices by cutting back on work and social activities. Despite these sacrifices, the majority (60 per cent) continue to feel guilty that they are not doing enough, and 75 per cent feel they are not doing as well as the good old days (9, 29). This indicates that the compelling need to care runs deep, and that the myths serve to reinforce it.

Government Uses the Myths to Their Advantage

Since women make up the majority of caregivers, the myths are directed at them and put them on the defensive as they push themselves to emulate a past that never existed. Despite massive evidence that the golden era of caregiving never existed, the myths refuse to die because, according to Brody (9), the guilt won't die. Women like Rebecca continue to feel guilty that they have failed their parents by not always being there for them. Value-laden words like 'dumping' and 'abandonment' are still used, and reinforce the myths. Elders help to uphold the myths by claiming abandonment, when all that has really happened is that their roles have changed with time. Governments are increasingly guilty of pushing the myths in an effort to save health care dollars. They maintain that family values have weakened and that the government is now providing most of the services and care for the elderly. They balk at providing universal daycare. They call for more community care (translation: women's unpaid caring). Yet studies show over and over again that the vast majority of caregiving is already being done by family members, most of them women like Rebecca (9, 29, 32).

Women like Rebecca must learn to ignore the myths and actively fight to destroy them. They must also learn to ask for help, and realize that it should not always have to be women who do all the caregiving: men must become more involved.

CHAPTER FIVE

Sharing the Caring with Family

'We can't go tomorrow night,' I said, struggling to keep the frustration out of my voice. I was cooking burgers on the hibachi for dinner, and Bryan was lounging in a chair in a rare moment of peace.

He looked up at me as if I'd stepped in something unmentionable.

'What do you mean we can't go? We've saved and planned for this for a month. A movie, quiet dinner for two. Our lunch last week wasn't exactly relaxing, you know.'

What an understatement, I thought. I'd been late from Peter's game and had had to gobble lunch in order to get back in time for work. It had been most unsatisfying, and I'd forgotten to bring some drinks to go with the sandwiches I'd made. But what could I say? We had obligations to others, too. Obligations that seemed more immediate, if not more important.

'Danielle's made the finals of the public speaking contest at the school and they're tonight at eight. She told me this morning. She only found out herself last night. We can't not go, Bryan.' We looked at each other, and I added: 'She leaves next week for Europe.'

Bryan sighed, then said –

'We can have an early dinner, then, and arrive a bit late. We don't have to listen to all the speeches.'

'No go, Bryan. Sorry.' I was furious with myself for having made new plans after work. 'I have an office meeting at five and I promised Dad I'd bring over our old TV after that because theirs just died and they want to see a show tonight. Mum also asked me to pick up some special cheese and some whipping cream.

Bryan's jaw dropped to his boots.

'Whipping cream? TV? Good God, Rebecca. Your mother does not *need* whipping cream. She may *want* it but she sure as hell doesn't *need* it, and our old TV is as dead as theirs.'

'It is?'

'Yes, and your father knows it. I told him this morning. I guess he just forgot.'

I saw him hesitate as if thinking twice about what he wanted to say, but his frustration got the better of him.

'Rebecca, this is the third time in a week we've had to rearrange our plans because of your parents or one of our kids. Why should they always get priority? When is it *our* turn, Rebecca? Look at us, for God's sake. We're getting old. What about your sisters and brother? Why can't *they* help with your parents?'

I remained silent, trying to collect my thoughts.

'Nowhere is it written that just one sister has to do it all. No matter how much you love your parents, there's a limit. Doesn't it bother you that they don't do anything to help out? Have you ever thought to ask them why they don't?'

'Of course it bothers me, but it just seems to have fallen on me to do it all.'

'Well make it fall on someone else sometimes.'

* * *

How Are Souciaires Chosen by Their Families?

That Rebecca has been 'chosen' by her siblings to be the primary souciaire for her parents is not unusual. Most families tend to 'choose' a sister or brother, who takes over most of the caregiving of parents. The remaining siblings then operate as secondary souciaires, ideally providing help when and as needed (1).

Naturally, if you are an only child or are the only sibling who lives within commuting distance of your parents, it will be assumed that you will be the one to take on the role of primary souciaire.

There are many factors that help predict who will become primary souciaire. As discussed in previous chapters, gender determines to a great degree who will provide the care. If you are female your chances of becoming a souciaire are far greater (1).

Some families choose the person with the fewest responsibilities to take on caregiving. Unmarried, widowed, or separated sons and daughters are expected to take on more responsibilities for elder care than their married counterparts. Indeed, all three generations expect more of unmarried sons and daughters than married ones. An unmarried sister with no children may appear to be less tied down than her sister with two kids, and so may be viewed as the obvious primary souciaire. But she may not like being tied down, or she may travel a lot and throw the ball back in her sister's court by saying, 'You're already tied down so it'll be easier for you.' Almost half of all daughters who provide elder care are unmarried (1). For some unmarried women, having someone to care for fills a basic human need – to be close to someone else. It provides them with an important role and with a warm relationship. Also, they find the role easier to take on, as they have no competing demands other than work. Indeed, such women often say that they consider elder care their responsibility because they have fewer other commitments (1).

Choosing an unmarried sibling to be primary souciaire can be taken to extreme lengths. One daughter living in Canada had an elderly widowed father living in Denmark. When it came time for him to need care, as he approached ninety years of age, she was expected to provide his care despite two sons living in the same city as their father. Their rationale, including the father's, was that the sons were both married and worked full time while the daughter, while fully employed, was not married. They felt she should come home and care for the father, but she liked her job and was happy in her new country. She became a long-distance primary care souciaire, which soon became unworkable as medical emergencies arose and her father needed immediate care. The sons suggested he move to Canada to be near the daughter, but after a lifetime in Denmark he wisely felt it would not make him happy. His children arranged for paid help (2).

The strongest incentive for helping elderly parents is the perception that they need help, and this appears to be the strongest predictor of caregiving. Caring for elders is an extension of what has taken place in the past (3). Usually, over the years one daughter responds to any crises, and keeps in touch. The relationship is usually mutually gratifying, and the souciaire votes herself in. For some this can happen precipitously as a previously autonomous parent suddenly gets ill; in Rebecca's case, which is more typical, the care expanded so gradually that no one noticed, to the point where suddenly she was the principal souciaire. Some souciaires volunteer prematurely, and in so doing accelerate the elder's dependence. Souciaires should ask themselves whether they are volunteering to satisfy their *own* needs rather than their parents'*actual* needs.

The child who gets along best with the parents may be elected by her siblings, or the parents, or both. One daughter said she understood her mother best and had always been a close friend while her sisters and brother had a more difficult relationship. It is much easier to care for someone when the personalities mesh.

A child perceived to be favoured over her siblings may take on the souciaire role because it is expected, or because she never felt she deserved the favoured role and wants to prove she does. She may take it on out of guilt at receiving so much attention.

The least favoured child may take on the caregiving role to gain approval. Sometimes a child who felt parental rejection does the caring in an attempt to displace a more loved sibling. Such children try to win acceptance by working themselves to the bone. Resentment can build if things don't work out and the elder is still seen as loving another child more, even when that is only a perception, and not the reality.

Some souciaires may volunteer in order to fulfil an unconscious need to be wanted. They have never cut the umbilical cord, and they sacrifice everything for their elders. They cannot stand having anyone else do the caring. They feel that their siblings would not know what to do; some actually refuse help even when they desperately need it. One woman who cared for her elderly mother couldn't leave the house. When her sister offered to come for a few days, she declined the offer because she felt her mother would not like it.

For these women, caregiving offers a role, a job, a sense of belonging. If they get approval for what they do, their self-esteem soars. These women are professional souciaires who go out of their way to establish their role. They may say the stress is unbearable and emotionally exhausting, but they make no effort to get help of any kind, and they neglect their own needs.

Souciaires to Parents-in-Law

Even when the elders are the husband's parents, it is likely the wife who will do most of the daily care. Often this is because the husband is an only child, or none of the other siblings live nearby. Some women simply assume the role once the caregiving falls to the husband, so deeply engrained is the notion that it is their job. In fact, many are grateful for any help they get from their husbands. They receive less help from their husbands than their brothers would from their wives in similar circumstances (1).

Most daughters-in-law feel less emotional involvement and experience less guilt when dealing with in-laws (unless the in-laws live in). They don't get as upset, and don't feel the same responsibility. Some daughters-in-law are very angry at having to care for in-laws and have no natural bond. Missing is the powerful motive of childhood ties, as in 'She took care of me, now I'll take care of her.' A daughter-in-law tends to do it for her husband, and must learn to involve him more. She should remember that her husband should have a greater incentive to help than she does; after all, by helping, he helps not only his parents but his wife as well (1).

It is wise to remember that it is often difficult to transfer the primary caregiving role to another once a pattern has been established. Don't take on the job simply to curry favour or out of guilt, fear, or anger. If these are your feelings, involve your brothers and sisters right from the start to see if someone else is better suited or wants to be primary souciaire. Also, ask why the bulk of the care should have to be provided by one person.

* * *

Bryan was right, of course – it was crazy not to rely on my sisters more, but they both had responsibilities of their own and I hated to ask them. I guess I had hoped they would ask me if I needed any help, but so far they hadn't. It took me most of the day to find both the resolve and the time to phone Heather, my eldest sister, at the factory where she worked. As I asked my question, I could hear in the background the clatter of heavy machinery.

'Whipping cream? Are you serious, Rebecca? You want me to take time off work to bring Mum some whipping cream?'

Phrased like that, it *did* sound ridiculous. I should have told her about the doctor's appointment, but she always made me nervous, and as soon as I heard her voice I'd just blurted out the first thing that came to my head. She always had that effect on me.

'Come on, Rebecca. It's got to be something more than that, surely. Is something wrong with Mum and Dad you're not telling me?'

'No, no,' I said hurriedly. 'It's just that I seem to have less and less time to do the little things they need done. You know, Dad's not as mobile as he used to be and I've been getting their groceries for them lately and helping out around the house and chauffeuring them when they need to see the doctor.'

'You've been buying the groceries? I thought Mum did that.' I heard the note of concern in her voice.

'Not without a car she can't. And she has an appointment tomorrow to see a doctor. She's been feeling really tired lately but I can't drive her. My boss will have a fit if I take more time off.'

'Why didn't you say so in the first place? It's a far sight better than whipping cream.'

A loud crash came down the phone line, and I heard her whispering to someone.

'Look, Rebecca, I can't help you tonight. It's just too short notice. I'm on night shift today and tomorrow.'

'That's just it, Heather – it's usually short notice and I need help. I can't always be the one to drop everything anymore. Do you think Sharon could do it?' Sharon was my kid sister.

'But she's got two toddlers at home,' Heather said impatiently. 'She'd have to bundle them into the car and then carry them into the doctor's. I don't see that as an option. Surely you can do it, Becca. You're closer to Mum than any of us and you live closer to them too. It's natural for you to do it. You've always been the one to help out in emergencies. When Dad fell, you took over. It just naturally seems to have fallen to you.'

'But I can't do it *all*, Heather.' I could hear the frustration in my voice but I couldn't do anything to hide it. There was a pause, and then she said in her big-sister voice –

'Look, surely you can take time off work this time around and we can talk if it happens again. Maybe you're overreacting. Mum and Dad don't need that much help, and maybe you're just spoiling them.' I heard someone else's voice in the background, and then, 'Look, I gotta go. Call me. We can talk.'

I carefully replaced the receiver and started dialling Sharon's number, but my heart wasn't in it – what would she be able to do with two toddlers? I cut the connection before it began to ring.

*   *   *

How Much Help Do Souciaires Get from Their Siblings?

The simple truth, backed up by research, is that most souciaires receive little if any help from their siblings. In one representative study, 65 per cent of souciaires said relatives helped, 4 per cent said they received only minimal help, and 31 per cent said they received no help at all; also, 40 per cent were not satisfied with the help they were receiving (4). Another study showed that when siblings live close to each other, the primary souciaire does 24 hours per week of care, but her sisters do eight and her brothers less than four (1).

Yet in many cases secondary souciaires may be helping more than the research indicates. Most studies look only at daily help and ignore help that is forthcoming during crisis. Most souciaires know they can count on their siblings or friends in times of crisis or to help with major tasks such as moving a parent. Also, souciaires have confirmed in studies (sparse as they are) that the emotional support they receive from siblings is extremely important (1). The knowledge that there is someone who can take over for you if you have to leave or get ill is very comforting; this applies not only to elder caregiving but to child care as well. Siblings, particularly sisters, can provide tremendous support to each other. They can give and receive advice, and they can offer to house a niece or nephew who is rebelling toward the parents or who needs a place to stay while attending school away from home. Advice about raising cildren, from infancy to adolescence to young adulthood, is often worth seeking and gladly given, and siblings, especially those who have been that route, can provide this as well. But it's not all roses.

How do sibling relationships affect caregiving? Is the souciaire able to ask for help? Does she want to? What problems are likely to arise?

Sibling Rivalry and Other Conflicts Causing Stress for Souciaires

Since caregiving responsibilities are often placed on one family member, there can be arguments right at the outset over who will do the caring. A souciaire may be loved for taking on the role and be well supported by siblings, or she may be hated for it. One woman used her parents as pawns in a lifelong power struggle over her sisters. Taking complete control over the care of the parents left her sisters with no say. Another woman used her position as primary souciaire to get even with her brother, whom she felt had always been treated better by her parents. She prevented her brother from developing the closer relationship he had always wanted with his parents by making it difficult for him to visit often or to take his parents on outings. Since the elders were living with their daughter, the son was powerless to do much about it. Some souciaires who help out their parents financially may use this fact to wield power over any siblings who contribute less.

As the needs of elders increase, so too do the stresses on sibling relationships. Sibling rivalry is never far below the surface. You will need to cope with the different ways that siblings view the care of their parents, and you will need to find ways of sharing equitably so as not to reinforce old family patterns. Remember that old loyalties and rivalries can resurface; also, that sibling relationships do not begin with parent care but are on a continuum, and that adjustments will need to be made related to sharing the caregiving.

There can be serious conflict or relatively little depending on

your family. That being said, one of the biggest complaints souciaires make is that they don't get enough help. Rebecca has felt
this, and indirectly so has Bryan. Souciaires see the inequity more
clearly as elders' needs rise, and are sensitive to the lack of help
from siblings. A sister may never forgive her siblings if she does it
all and they never help. Arguments over who does more can lead
to tension, hostility, rivalry, jealousy, and resentment.

One common source of strain on souciaires is a sibling who pre-
tends to be a major souciaire but delegates everything. Example: A
sister does all the day-to-day caregiving, and then the brother
breezes in and takes his parents out for an outing and they live on
it for weeks. The sister is doing the everyday chores, which everyone is taking for granted. She resents the fact that her brother
gives her parents special treats while she helps them live.

Another source of stress for souciaires is the criticism and unsolicited advice their siblings proffer concerning the care they are
providing. This can be quite demoralizing, especially in light of the
fact that according to one study, two-fifths of primary souciaires
said their parents favoured another sibling (1). The favoured sibling may have more influence over the parents; as a result, any
advice he gives that contradicts the primary souciaire may cause
problems. One son took his mother out for dinner, and told her
that the sugar-free diet his sister had put the mother on was way
too strict and suggested she order anything she wanted. It was his
sister who ended up caring for her diabetic mum when she got ill.

One son suggested that his mother might like to change to his
family doctor. This was enough for the mother to ask her daughter
to make an appointment and drive her there. Understandably, the
daughter was furious with the brother in view of the fact that the
mother's doctor was excellent, knew the mother's medical history
well, and lived close by. But once the suggestion was raised, the
mother insisted on changing doctors.

Another daughter criticized a retirement home picked out by
her sister and accepted by the parents, though she had never even
seen it. This undermined the parents' confidence in the home,
and they changed their minds.

Another son, who never provided any sort of care because he

lived in another city, came to visit one day and criticized his sister about the nursing home she had chosen for their father, implying that things would have been different had he been around. No one likes to be criticized, but somehow it seems worse if you are criticized for doing something to help someone else. Siblings who criticize the care their sister is giving can undermine the entire caregiving process. One sister, who lived in another city, came to visit her parents and criticized her sister for letting her father gain so much weight. Souciaires are often criticized for how their elders look, or dress, or for their living conditions. They can be criticized for visiting too little, or being too pushy, or not finding the right doctor quickly enough. All of this is very demoralizing when the critic is doing nothing to help at all.

It may be well-intentioned advice or concern, but that doesn't mean it is constructive. 'Is the doctor really OK?' is not the sort of question a souciaire wants to hear when she has gone to great lengths to get the best she can but is aware that medical science can only do so much. Being reminded of the negatives can be depressing, and can freeze souciaires with indecision. If you are primary souciaire, you can avoid such scenarios by involving your siblings in all plans and making sure they know the medical status of your elders. The alternative is to listen to a lot of unwarranted criticism from back-seat souciaires.

Suggestions for Sharing the Caring

For a primary souciaire, the objective is to spread the caregiving around until the point is reached where *no one* is the primary souciaire because *everyone* is chipping in to help. Some siblings, usually sisters, do this by collaborating. In one case, one sister took over the medical and bureaucratic chores while the other dealt with hands-on care. The arrangement was seen by both as fair sharing rather than equal sharing, as it suited their personalities. It makes no sense to ask a sibling who is terrified of the telephone to take on a search for services when she would be better suited to doing the accounting.

How do your siblings perceive the situation? If they have never helped before, it may not occur to them to help now. Don't be a martyr: it helps no one. Everyone likes to help to some extent, and by denying your siblings that pleasure you scare them away. If you have brothers or sisters, tell them what you need. Ask them to help. Don't wait for them to ask, as they may be deferring to you as primary souciaire and believe you don't need much, if any, help because you have said nothing. Give them a chance to help by suggesting something they can do.

Gather them together and map out a plan of what the various needs are and who will do what and when. Air out any problems. Keep the meeting open and flexible and avoid confrontation. Include your elders in these discussions. Will they accept help from other siblings? If not, why not? What sort of help do they need, and how can you divide up the tasks? Look at everyone's strengths and their likes, and then dislikes, and then try to divide the chores accordingly.

It helps to write a list of all the help that is needed so that siblings can get an idea of what you have been doing. Be specific about defining the tasks; describe how long they take, how often they must be done, and where they are carried out. A daily schedule may be the best approach, to show all the work that must be done and point out where others can be of assistance. Get your family to sign up for some of the tasks, and avoid the 'you' word (as in 'You never do anything'). Instead, use the 'I' word, for example, 'I need some help,' and 'I feel tired and stressed.' Let them know how being the primary souciaire is affecting you. Avoid laying blame. Get a sibling or an adult child to take over for a week or a month. Or, if you are caring for parents at home, ask your siblings to come and stay with your parents while you go away.

When Elders Live with the Souciaire

It is important for souciaires and their siblings to understand the special circumstances revolving around elders who live with the souciaire. Siblings usually contribute even less if the primary souciaire is caring for her elders in her own home; the usual assumption here is that things are now easier for the souciaire. After all, many

chores are done for the household as a whole – shopping, cleaning, and laundry are extended to the elder but are not much more
of a burden. Siblings thus may believe that the souciaire's needs
are being met, and the souciaire herself may rationalize that most
chores would have to be done anyway. After all, buying an extra
pork chop or doing an extra load of laundry is not as onerous as
having to shop and deliver groceries to elders living alone.

But siblings should continue to help by visiting, offering respite
care, and taking parents on outings. They should remember that
parents being cared for in the home tend to have disabilities,
whereas parents being cared for outside the home probably are
much better able to help themselves. In the same vein, souciaires
must communicate their needs to their siblings and delegate or ask
them to do various tasks. Rebecca has not even bothered to let her
sisters know that she's been doing the grocery shopping. She
should suggest they phone regularly to ask what they can do. If
they don't, she should phone them.

The Stresses Felt by Secondary Souciaires: Brothers and Sisters

It isn't only the primary souciaire who feels the strain of caregiving; souciaires must be aware of their siblings' feelings, and vice
versa. Very little research has been conducted on how siblings
interact with one another over parent care. Researchers tend to
hear only second-hand, from the souciaires, what their siblings are
feeling and doing. This lack of firsthand information leaves the
door open for all kinds of interpretations and misinterpretations,
such as, 'They're getting off scot free,' and 'They're having an easy
ride.' This is a recipe for creating guilty siblings – especially sisters.

One study showed that sisters are very sensitive about suggestions that they are not meeting their elders' needs; also, they tend
to feel more guilt than their brothers, and the primary souciaire
about not doing more, or not spending enough time with their
parents (1). They can only alleviate their guilt by doing something.
They are much more uncomfortable in the role of secondary souciaire than are their brothers, who generally are less involved with
elder care and feel the least strain. Sisters complained more than

brothers about being made to feel guilty about not doing enough. Brothers of the primary souciaire tend to provide only sporadic help, and their sisters see this as inadequate to meet the ongoing needs of parents (1).

It is more common for sons to be seen as unreliable in providing help. This is often accepted without question; yet a daughter who can't be counted on is either criticized, or apologized for, or made the target of much anger. This simply reinforces the view that women should be the souciaires (1).

The same study showed that secondary souciaires are not immune from caregiver's stress. About 50 per cent of secondary souciaires experience some of the same problems as the primary souciaire. These include emotional symptoms such as nervousness, frustration, and tiredness, and the strain of having their lives inter-rupted and marriages affected. Once again, things divide along gender lines, with sisters feeling more strain than brothers. A last point here: sisters feel good when allowed to share decisions about their parents (1).

Sisters feel more guilt than brothers about living too far away to help, and are more likely to want to move closer. They also report more negative feelings and more problems with siblings. Sisters are more likely than brothers to complain about being made to feel guilty, or being told they don't know what their mother wants, or being criticized for the help they give. They often feel left out, helpless, cut off, and uninformed, and worry about being able to arrive in good time when needed. They also worry about not being able to assert themselves in decision making because they do not do the caring (1).

Call that family meeting and involve your siblings!

*   *   *

It was Saturday morning, my one day to sleep in. The phone rang loudly by the bed, and I pulled my pillow over my ears, trying to block it out. We'd driven Danielle to the airport the night before and had had an emotional goodbye. I was still recovering from the shock of seeing my daughter leave home. It was 7 a.m. Someone else could answer it. I was sleeping in.

The ringing finally stopped, and I heard Bryan's muffled voice –
'Calm down. I can't hear you. You're talking too fast.'

Puzzled, I relaxed my grip on the pillow and let it roll off my
head and land on the floor to the side of the bed. I caught the look
of concern spreading like a stain across Bryan's face, and my heart
turned cold with fear.

'We'll meet you at the hospital,' he said, and my heart lunged.

He hung up and said quickly, 'I think it's OK, Becca, but your
Dad thinks your mother's either had a stroke or a heart attack.
She's apparently alert, though, which is a good thing.'

'Where's Dad? Is he with her?'

'Yeah. He went in the ambulance. She wouldn't go without him.
He wants you to bring some clothes and things for her.'

I looked at him in some kind of wild appeal.

He gave me a big hug and said, 'It's going to be OK, Rebecca.
Your Mum's tough – she'll pull through.'

But all I could think of was how awful she'd looked the other day
and how I hadn't done anything about it. Maybe I was being too
hard on myself. After all, how could I have known?

Bryan was right. Mum was tough, but it took all she had to deal
with the disabilities caused by a mild stroke. Although the stroke
hadn't affected her speech or memory, she was partially paralysed
on her left side. The doctors said we were looking at a hospital stay
of maybe two months, including rehab.

What was almost more alarming was my father. I was stunned at
just how much my mother had been doing to care for him. Even
with my regular visits to their little bungalow, I hadn't realized just
how much he depended on my mother. When I picked him up to
take him to visit Mum, he always told me he didn't need anything.
The day after Mum went into hospital, I'd stocked his fridge for
him with easy-to-cook meals. He was always waiting outside for me
when I came to pick him up, and always insisted I just drop him off
when we returned.

But one day he forgot his wallet and asked me to nip up and get
it. When I opened the front door it was partly jammed by a pile of
unread newspapers and junk mail. There were dozens of dirty cups
and empty tin cans in the sink, and the laundry was piled high.

There were piles of garbage out on the back porch stairs and the racoons had got into it. His medications stood untouched on the kitchen table, and the fridge was more or less still full: even the milk, which by some miracle had not yet soured, stood untouched.

'Dad, why didn't you ask me for help?' I asked him as I handed him his wallet.

He looked at me, genuinely surprised. 'I don't need any help.' He didn't seem to care – he just missed my mother.

'But the newspapers – can't you carry them upstairs?' I imagined him trying to manage the two steps with his walker while carrying the newspaper and the mail. Of course Mum would have carried them up for him.

He looked at me and shrugged. 'Not much use to me without your mother.'

Puzzled, I asked him what he meant.

'I can't read the papers anymore, the print's too small – my eyes aren't good enough. Your mother always reads the important parts to me, but even she needs a magnifying glass now, if it isn't the big print.' He was surprised I didn't know. So was I. No wonder he listened to Beethoven so much.

'And the fridge – it's still full of food. What have you been eating?'

'I'm fine, Rebecca, just fine. I'm simply not as hungry as I used to be.'

'But Dad, you and Mum went through that much food in four days.'

He shrugged.

He didn't seem to mind or even notice the mess. It was obvious that Mum had been the one to keep everything neat, tidy, and clean, and that Dad hadn't thought much about it. He hadn't asked for help because he really didn't need help – he'd never done the cleaning up. When I came in and did it for him he didn't consider it as help. It was a real eye-opener for me.

I was worried about him and unsure what to do. He was obviously having trouble getting dressed in the morning because his clothes were always dishevelled, and I suspected he was also having trouble bathing. But I didn't know what to do about it. Mum was worried sick and asked me to do something.

I called my sisters, and after much arguing and jostling of egos over many days we divided up the work among us as best we could: the shopping, the meals, the transportation to medical appointments, and the housecleaning. I'd even got Dad to agree to pay a handyman to come twice a month to help him with his tiny garden. But one day we had a crisis: Heather was away on business, Sharon had two sick toddlers, and my whole family was sick with the flu. Dad needed to go to the doctor's for an appointment he had waited months for, and no one could take him. When I phoned him from bed and suggested he splurge on a taxi, he refused, point blank, saying he couldn't afford it. When I offered to pay for it he changed the subject.

'What about your brother, Rebecca?' asked Bryan as he blew his nose and hunkered down beside me in bed. 'Where does it say it has to be just sisters? What about Matthew? You've let him off the hook scot free.'

'He's got an important job, Bryan. I can't ask him to miss work.'

'Why on earth not? *You* miss work. Your career is just as important as his. Your sister misses work and your other sister has to juggle her toddlers. For God's sake, *I've* even missed work, and much as I love them they're not even my parents. I'm surprised at you, Becca – in this new world of equal opportunity you're letting your brother off the hook. Why can't you three bring yourselves to ask your brother to help?'

Three days later Bryan found me moping in the living room. He came and gave me a hug and asked what was up.

'Matthew.'

'What about him? Did you ask him to help out?'

'Yes, and he said he would.'

'Terrific.'

'No, not terrific. First he got his wife to do the stuff, but I pointed out that was unfair to her and so now on the days he's supposed to get groceries he's hired someone to deliver them. Lucky him – he can afford to do that. On the day he was supposed to help, all he did was stop by after work for a chat. That's all he did – no housework, nothing, just a chat.'

'What's wrong with that, if he can afford it? Your father got a nice, uninterrupted visit.'

I glared at him and said –

'That's not all. He was supposed to take Dad to see Mum, too, but instead he paid a chauffeur service to do it.'

'So?'

'So Dad's not a parcel to be delivered by strangers!'

'You're just miffed because he refused to take that taxi the other day and now here he is happily accepting Matthew's chauffeur service. Did he complain?'

I hesitated. 'No, not really. He actually seemed to enjoy all the fuss over which chauffeur service was the best. But that still doesn't mean it's OK. We can't afford what Matthew can, and it makes us look cheap.'

'Look, Rebecca,' said Bryan slowly. 'Everyone has their own way of looking after their loved ones. I happen to agree with Matthew. If you can afford to buy the help for things like cleaning and shopping and even chauffeuring, why ever not, especially if you're the only person who can care for them? Why burn yourself out on the physical stuff when you can spend your time visiting, not dusting?'

'Wouldn't that make you feel guilty, if it were *your* father we were talking about?'

'No. Why should it?'

I stared at him and marvelled that men and women actually belonged to the same species. Maybe there were some things I could learn from the men in my life about different approaches to caregiving.

*   *   *

What Role Do Men Play in Caregiving?

Although most souciaires are women, a small but growing number of men are helping more than before, and women – including Rebecca – must actively seek out this resource. Unfortunately, to date women have been notorious for accepting men's tiny role in caregiving and excuse their husbands and brothers (as Rebecca is doing) without even thinking. They accept it as a given that men are not souciaires. Elders often reinforce their sons' excuses by refusing help from sons who are too busy or whose work they perceive as too important to interrupt. They then turn to a daughter, whose job may be just as important as her brother's, if not more so (1).

Some cultures make it virtually impossible for men to help, let alone be primary souciaire. In a study of Greek women, it was found that husbands expected their wives to do all the caregiving: it was frowned upon if men did such chores. The same was found among Lebanese women, who agreed with their husbands that men do not do housework (5). In view of Canada's growing multiculturalism, more research is needed into the cultural and ethnic values that dictate caregiving according to gender. Ethnic women cannot be expected to continue taking the entire burden as well as working full time, and men should not be denied the chance to help simply because it is 'frowned upon.'

Even in North America, research shows that the help men give tends to divide along gender lines. Women provide more emotional and nurturing help than do men, perhaps because of their past experience caring for children (6). In another study, both sexes saw men as less empathic to the needs of elders, and saw men's excuses for not taking on the primary caregiving role as more reasonable than women's, however ill-founded this might be (7). Men provide the concrete help in terms of finances, home repairs, and decision making. The day-to-day, hands-on care is still considered woman's work, and any emotional support is usually provided by sisters or wives. This makes it easier for men to feel less guilt, as it keeps them at a greater emotional distance than women when helping their parents. It also leaves the burden squarely, and unfairly, on the shoulders of women.

But there are changes in the wind. Twenty years ago, child care was very different from what it is today. More and more women now drive their toddlers to day care and ask their husbands to help. Husbands are responding by helping out with kids more than ever before. The same pattern is just beginning to take hold in elder care: more sons are carrying out more than just their traditional roles of banking and home repairs. Some are shopping, cooking, and cleaning, and a rare few are even providing personal care, especially to their fathers (shaving, bathing, and so on). However, men still leave personal care of their mothers to their wives (6).

More men are asking about where to get services, and at some hospitals as many men as women are bringing in elders for appointments and medical tests. A higher divorce rate could account for this: divorced men are suddenly having to care for elders whom their wives would have cared for in the past. But some of this is likely related to the fact that more women are working, and that more men see the need to pull their own weight in the caregiving arena.

Men as Souciaires

Men caring for their elders is not a sweeping trend, it may not even be a trend, and but it *is* a beginning. It's none too soon, for as we head into the twenty-first century more sons will have to take on the role of souciaire. Women have had enough of doing it all. With the increasing numbers of 'oldest' old (those older than eighty-five), more sons and daughters will be needed to provide care, since by definition the oldest old are at high risk for physical and mental disabilities and illnesses.

No one knows how many men provide most of the care for their elders or their spouses, but it is rare. One American study estimates that 9 per cent of sons care for their elders and that 13 percent of husbands look after their spouses (8). But even here, most men take on the role of primary souciaire only if there are no female relatives to take over, as in the case of being an only child or having only brothers. When they do take over care, usually their wives help them substantially. If they have neither wives or sisters, they generally buy the necessary care for their spouse or parents (1).

Men are more likely to become souciaires if they belong to the working class and thus lack the resources to buy care, or lack legitimate excuses to refuse to care (9). In sharp contrast, women are expected to care. People don't notice when sons don't do the caring – they only notice when they do. It is the reverse for women.

There have been very few studies on men as primary souciaires. Most studies of male souciaires have focused on husbands caring for wives, which is not surprising, since men are far more likely to provide both instrumental and personal care to their spouses than to anyone else (6).

Those few men who do provide total care for their elders and spouses, including personal care and hygiene, tend to provide similar care as women, and at roughly the same frequency. One study showed that men provide 10.9 hours of care per week versus 11.8 for women in identical situations (9). Though still rare, it is more common to see a man provide hands-on care for his wife than for his parents, particularly his mother. A recent study found that those rare men who do provide total care for their elders or spouses tend to be more compassionate and emotionally 'warmer' than other men (6).

Most of the 148 male souciaires in this study were over sixty. All were caring for their wives. It was found that these men saw themselves as possessing traits normally more common among women: compassionate, warm, and gentle as opposed to competitive, aggressive, and forceful. The same study found that it was easier for men to care for someone if they possessed these former traits.

Differences in How Men and Women Provide Care

Most men who take on the role of primary souciaire do not provide personal care. By and large they handle care differently from women, as Rebecca is discovering with her brother Matthew. Sons and husbands who are souciaires are not as likely to sacrifice anything in order to provide care. Sons, like Matthew, are more likely to *manage* the care for their elders or their spouses as opposed to actually providing hands-on care themselves (10). They view their careers as important and look for a balance that does not force them to choose between career and care. Thus, sons and husbands tend to use formal services more often and to resort to those services sooner than daughters and wives. They spend their time organizing care and sorting out problems on the phone, and the time they actually spend with their parents or spouses revolves around outings and visits. They do not seem to feel the same guilt or concern over their parents' or spouse's feelings as do women; they also find it easier to buy services for them and, if the time comes, to arrange a good retirement or nursing home without being consumed by guilt.

Most women tend to be care providers unless they are among the minority who, like their brothers or husbands, view their own careers as important. Then, like their male folk, they manage the care of their parents or husband instead of providing that care personally. These women are under less strain than care providers, who tend to have less education, to be less career oriented, to hold jobs that are less valued by society, and to lack the money to buy care (11).

Research has shown that men are better at recognizing their own needs and meeting them while still caring for elders or a spouse. For example, husbands do not expect their wives' needs to interfere with their own ongoing projects, such as gardening or carpentry; also, they have no difficulty leaving a spouse at home alone or deciding what is best for her. In contrast, women give priority to the care recipients' needs and take pains to include them in decisions and allow them choices. Women find it more difficult than men to take over control of their spouse's care and to deal with the spouse's anger in a caregiving situation. They also worry more. Generally, men are more used to having power and to making decisions; they simply take over caregiving, and the decisions associated with it, as a natural progression stemming from their work and their decision-making role in the family. Women do learn over time to cope, and it has been suggested that this is because they learn to distance themselves emotionally – a strategy men use frequently (7).

The help provided by sons decreases when the sons get a job or when they marry, but daughters do not decrease their help in similar circumstances. Men are less likely than women to use sick days to help elders; they are also less likely to miss work related to social events because of their obligations as souciaires. Men report fewere losses of career opportunities related to turning down or not seeking promotion. However, men who provide personal care are more likely to report workplace and personal costs than men who don't provide personal care (9).

* * *

We'd got down to a pretty good routine, with Heather, Matthew, Sharon, and I taking turns stopping in on Dad and fixing supper, but I'd had a bad day at work and, as luck would have it, it was my turn to help him.

I pulled into the driveway after work, my head screaming bloody murder, and went straight to the fridge for a cool drink. I figured I had ten minutes to relax before having to get up and do the errands.

I was lying on the sofa feeling sorry for myself when I heard Bryan's footsteps. I wondered why he was home so early. He literally bounced into the living room.

'What are you looking so downcast about?' he asked.

'Don't ask,' I said miserably.

He waved thrcc tickets in my face, did a pirouette, and landed flat on his rear end. I was so far gone I could only manage a tiny smile until he told me what he was waving in my face.

'Tickets to the baseball game,' he announced, a grin splitting his face.

I couldn't believe it! We hadn't gone to a game in years because the price of the tickets had gone up so much, and we didn't know any well-heeled people with season's tickets to spare.

'When?' I asked eagerly, sitting up, my headache miraculously vanishing.

'Tonight, and a nice long quiet intimate dinner afterwards. Just for you and I.'

My smile froze on my face, even as I resisted the urge to correct his grammar.

'But tonight is my night to –'

Bryan interrupted with a laugh.

'Your Dad knows already. He got the tickets from an old friend who owed him a favour. Figured you and I needed a break.'

'But what is he going to do about dinner and stuff? I can't ask Heather or Sharon or Matthew, and he really can't get it himself, and he doesn't like having strangers come in.'

Bryan thumbed the tickets and smiled again. 'David and Peter have it all worked out. He's in good hands and so are they.'

'David and Peter?' I asked in disbelief.

He laughed. 'We haven't been completely deaf to your appeals for help, you know.'

I felt a nice, warm, delicious feeling stealing through my body like the warmth of a fire on a cold night. People cared about *me!* About *us!* But then I eyed him suspiciously and said –

'Why are there *three* tickets?'

He laughed and said, 'When I picked up the tickets I got suckered in by a cute little kid selling raffle tickets for some charity. First prize, all expenses paid weekend trip to ...'

With a flourish he handed me the ticket.

'... to Montreal, including an Expos game and a night on the town in the Old City. We can pretend it's Paris if we win and dance into the wee hours ...'

What a hopeless romantic, I thought as he offered me his arm and bowed dramatically to the floor. 'Shall we go?' he asked, his eyebrows cocked in wild exaggeration. I laughed as we waltzed out of the living room en route to the ball game.

*   *   *

Help from Husbands

Research suggests that husbands play a minimal role in helping their wives with caregiving (12, 1). So deeply ingrained is the nurturing role that married daughters do not expect much (if anything) from their husbands in terms of day-to-day help. Indeed, many souciaires describe their husbands as being supportive if they simply refrain from criticizing or interfering with caregiving. Recent research indicates that the single most important support husbands provide their wives is emotional support. Wives value it and consider it more important than any physical help. When caregiving becomes too demanding, the husband can be a calming influence. If elders criticize how care is given, or if the children demand too much, the husband makes a good sounding board for the souciaire, an emotional well from which she can draw strength and support. Physical and financial help is also a big plus, and many wives who are souciaires say they could not have done it all without their husband (7, 13, 14).

It is not surprising, therefore, that married daughters generally feel less stress and strain than unmarried daughters when caring for their parents. The emotional support of a husband or partner and children can do a great deal to counteract some of the negatives, such as competition for time, which can cause souciaires so much stress. Married souciaires talk about both the positives of being married while caregiving, and the negatives. One woman, when asked who had the hardest time in terms of caregiving and marital status, answered 'married women' – and then gave the same answer when asked who had the easiest time (1).

Husbands under Strain

A recent study showed that most men find that caregiving by wives neither hurts nor helps their marriage; wives are more likely to say that it causes disruptions (14). Most souciaires report that caregiving does not harm their marriage (14, 15, 16).

Husbands of souciaires do report that they are often under strain. Yet the stresses they report are usually related to their own losses. They are bothered by the lifestyle restrictions that caregiving imposes. A large minority report irritants such as interference with their own plans, work interruptions, a lack of time for themselves, and a loss of time with their wives. However, these stresses are the result of their *wives*, not themselves, providing care (5, 7).

Husbands are well aware of the problems facing their wives – more so if the elders are living with them – and many see their wives as being caught between their parents and their husbands and kids. Those whose wives are caring for disabled elders see the burden on their wives as greater than what the wives themselves feel (1).

Ask the Men in Your Life to Help

Involve your husband as an equal player. Emotional support is great, but hands-on help would make things even better. If you are caring for his parents, get him to share the care by outlining what you need and expect from him. Don't serve him with ultimatums, but have suggestions on hand and talk them over with a view to finding a better balance. The old excuse – 'It's easier for me to do the laundry, the food shopping, the driving ...' – results in you doing it all. It may take a while for your husband to learn to do some of the chores, if he hasn't done them before, but persevere: it's past time.

If it is *your* parents that you are caring for, rather than his, the incentive for him to help out with them will be less. If it's nearly impossible to get him to help you with them then get him to help you with chores around the house to ease your burden. By doing the grocery shopping and cooking dinner for the family – from both of which he will benefit directly – he will be giving you more opportunity to help your parents and still be there for your family.

Elders and Children Provide Help Too

Don't ever forget as helpers the very people for whom you are caring: elders and children. Both can and do contribute enormously to the caregiving experience. By the very nature of life, those who receive care and are unable to give any in return are the very young and the very old. Elders who are physically or mentally disabled need a great deal of care, as do all infants and young children. Most of us fall somewhere in between, and both give and receive care. Elders who are more or less autonomous can give as much help as they receive, and often they give far more.

You may be finding that you are doing more for your parents in terms of grocery shopping and chauffeuring, and that they are more in need of care then before; but if you are really honest with yourself you may be surprised at just how much help your parents still give you. In fact, they are much more likely to give help than to receive it until they are among the 'oldest' old, at which point the balance shifts.

Grandparents help over the years by intermittently babysitting their grandchildren. A British study showed more than one-third of working mothers had their mothers or mothers-in-law babysit for them (17). Many grandmothers take pleasure in and do a great deal of babysitting for their sons and daughters. Others are more reluctant but can sometimes be called upon to babysit, or pick up the kids after school, or (if they themselves don't work) care for them when they are sick during the working week. Often the help is financial, with parents loaning money interest-free to their children or holding a mortgage on their home. Clearly, then, neither parent nor child should be seen as solely a giver of aid. Souciaires find companionship with their elders, and receive advice from them, and can share joys and disappointments with them. The durability of family relationships hinges on how well you treat your elders and on how well your elders treat you. People *like* to give. When elders perceive themselves as valued members of the family, their self-esteem is enhanced. Helping grandchildren is good for their morale.

Grandparents and Grandchildren Helping Each Other

Many grandparents keep in touch with their grandchildren, inviting them over for dinner, or helping them with school projects, or giving advice. When grandparents and grandchildren develop a relationship with each other, it helps the souciaire with both her parents and her children at the same time!

Grandparents, having been freed from the role of parenting, can indulge in a carefree relationship with their grandchildren. Sometimes the generation gap between grandparents and grandchildren is smaller than the one between parents and children because elders do not have the same responsibilities as parents toward the child. Some grandchildren find it easier to talk to their grandparents about emotional problems; as a result, grandparents can find themselves in the role of confidant. One grandparent was heard to say, 'If I'd known grandchildren were so much fun I would have had them first.' Grandparents can offer warmth and compassion and a shoulder to lean on, and in doing so help spread out the emotional work involved in raising children. More grandparents than ever before are picking up baseball glove and ball and throwing to their grandchildren, going biking with them, skiing or

playing tennis with them, reading to them, building and reinforc-
ing a lasting relationship. Also, they often offer financial support
in terms of educational expenses and a place to live during university and that first, difficult job search. They may even help a grandchild find a job.

You can help your children develop a good relationship with
their grandparents by encouraging them to visit, or to phone regularly. Plan outings together as a family. Teach your kids how to play
bridge and unleash them on your parents. Get them to help out.
Grandchildren say that parents are vital in helping build the relationship and that much depends on the parents' relationship with
their own parents.

One granddaughter who seldom saw her grandmother got a
phone call from her mother saying her grandmother, who was now
in a retirement home, missed her, and could she phone now and
again? The granddaughter, who was leading a busy married life
while working her way through university, could never find the
time to phone her grandmother during the day and early eve-
nings, and when she did have time she always assumed it was too
late at night. But the elderly often sleep less, or not as well. When
the grandmother phoned late one night (at 11:30), the two realized it was the ideal time, and from then on the granddaughter
phoned and they talked for half an hour every night. The relationship, once a rather distant one, blossomed overnight into a strong
and lasting one. What a loss it would have been had they not discovered a perfect time to talk on a daily basis. The conversation
involved the senior in her granddaughter's life and allowed the
granddaughter to gain advice and wisdom from her grandmother.
Both looked forward to these phone calls, which lightened the
caregiving burden of the primary souciaire, who saw needs being
met for both elder and child that otherwise might have had to be
met in some fashion by her.

Your adult and adolescent children can also share the care. In
the literature, adult and adolescent children are often viewed as
increasing the stress on their parents – especially the mother –
thereby making the souciaire role even more burdensome. They
are also seen as yet another source of competing demands for the

souciaire's time and energy. While this is true sometimes, it is usually not true at all times, and seldom so true as to make burnout likely. The positives prevail most of the time (14, 18, 19).

In one Canadian study, 83 per cent of souciaires said that having young adults at home was no hindrance, and 75 per cent said they helped. Only 21 per cent of souciaires said that older children didn't help (14). Grandchildren helped out the souciaire by visiting, shopping, cooking, cleaning, and doing errands. The older the grandchildren, the more help they provided, either directly to their grandparents or indirectly, by giving advice, encouragement, and support to the primary souciaire. Older grandchildren act as backup for the souciaire when needed, moving in to help in times of emergency and when asked. They provide a substantial amount of emotional support to souciaires, although their help is rarely counted in surveys and is therefore mostly invisible (20).

Grandchildren see their grandparents or contact them regularly. One representative study found that 35 per cent saw them daily, 14 per cent weekly, and 22 per cent at least once a month. Thirteen per cent of those living at a distance wrote or phoned weekly, while 22 per cent phoned or wrote monthly. In fact, grandchildren have personal contact with their grandparents as often as middle-aged sons and fathers have contact with each other (21).

Grandchildren feel that they have definite responsibilities toward their grandparents. A majority feel they should help when needed and should not expect money for helping. Also, a majority say they visit out of love, while 20 per cent say they visit because their parents did, and 11 per cent because it is expected. More and more grandchildren are becoming primary souciaires to their grandparents if their own parents are ill or unable to provide such care (22).

Some souciaires receive informal help from their parents' brothers and sisters. Siblings often come closer together again after their children have left home, even if they have lived separate lives. Although horizontal relationships are not much researched, there is no question that they exist, and primary souciaires should not ignore these as potential sources of informal help.

CHAPTER SIX

Formal Help Is on the Way

When I went to check on Dad a couple of days later and bring him some groceries, the gardener I had hired was angrily tossing his tools into his battered old van and muttering to himself. I could see Dad's pint-sized lawn was only half-cut, and I wondered what had happened now.

The gardener glared at me when I asked him why he was leaving. 'You just ask that old guy in there, lady. I'll not have anything more to do with him. I couldn't do anything right. Who does he think I am, anyway? I'll refund his damn money and you can find someone else.'

'Wait!' I protested, but he waved me away and tore off in his rusty van. It hadn't been easy finding someone to do the lawn at a cut-rate price.

'He wasn't any good anyway, Becca.'

I turned and saw Dad looking out the window at me.

'Look! He trampled my petunias and he insisted on coming right when I needed to nap, and besides his machine was terribly smelly, nearly killed me in my sleep, so I told him to leave. I don't need him anyway.'

'But Dad, you *do* need him.' Wrong, I thought – *I* need him.

'I'll get Peter to do it. He's a good lad and could use the money for a better barber. I'd rather pay him than some stranger, anyway.'

Why hadn't I thought of that in the first place? It was a good idea, and I was relieved that I wouldn't have to make a whole new set of phone calls to find someone else. I dumped the groceries in

the practically untouched fridge and saw the empty tins of maca-
roni lined up like little soldiers. Was that all he'd had to eat in the
last few days?

I glanced around at the pile of laundry, and the dust gathering
on the tables, and realized that Sharon must have been too busy
the day before to clean up. It wasn't the first time that had happened. We'd all been guilty of it more than once.

He'd followed me into the kitchen. I said in exasperation –

'Dad. I know you hate cooking, so why don't you let us arrange
for someone to come in with meals, and maybe do some other stuff
too.'

'You mean *strangers?* Inside my home?'

Mum and Dad had always been very private people, which is why
I had taken so long to bring up the subject.

'Well, yeah, but it's not as if they're going to spend the whole day
with you or take over your home. We can get Meals on Wheels to
bring some of your meals, and maybe get a housekeeper in to
clean the place at a reasonable price and help you out an hour a
day or so, and I'm sure there are lots of other options we can look
into that you could afford.'

He remained silent, and I continued, resisting the sudden
impulse to ask him to stay with us.

'That way, Dad, you can stay in your own home, and when Mum
comes back she won't feel she has to do all that work anymore.'

He stared at me, and our eyes locked as the implications of what
I had said sunk in. We both knew Mum wouldn't be able to do it all
anymore.

'I'll give it a try,' he said softly.

*   *   *

Services for Seniors Needing Some Help to
Remain in Their Own Home

Most elders prefer to remain in their own home for as long as possible and usually will take advantage of any help they can find in
order to do that. Dependence is relative: some elderly find that by
using services they become dependent on those services, but also

remain independent to a degree that would have been impossible otherwise. Many elders arrange for the services themselves and do not involve souciaires; more often, however, a son or daughter arranges for the services.

Across the country there is a wide range of nonprofit community support services geared to helping elders stay at home. These vary among communities, and some are not available everywhere.

Services include Meals on Wheels, which delivers two meals to the elder's home each day at noon from Monday to Friday, with extra meals to carry through the weekend. Anyone over sixty and living alone and unable to prepare meals is eligible. So are disabled adults. The maximum cost is about $5 per day; the actual amount charged may be much less than this depending on the elder's ability to pay. Wheels to Meals is a service that picks up elders and drives them to their meals Monday to Friday. Other services available for elders living at home include help with light housekeeping (vacuuming, dusting, laundry, and so on) and handyman services, which can include gardening work and snow removal as well as home maintenance and heavy-duty cleaning. Fees range from minimum wage to whatever the market can bear, depending on whether the service provider is a nonprofit or a commercial operation.

Various community services exist that allow elders to take advantage of group transportation to a shopping centre, or to give their shopping list to a volunteer, who will buy the groceries and deliver them. Elders can go shopping themselves with the help of a volunteer. Volunteer drivers can be arranged for transportation to and from medical appointments and other important engagements. Elders who live alone and feel uneasy about no one checking on them can sign on for a security check. Volunteers will phone or visit on a regular basis to make sure the elder is well and not in trouble. Many of these services are free where need can be demonstrated. Most provinces have financial assistance for elders needing medical devices such as wheelchairs, hearing aids, and walkers. Many areas of the country now have emergency systems: elders wear a transmitter with a push button; if they find themselves in trouble after falling, or fear they are ill, they can push the button and help will come, twenty-four hours a day. Check your Yellow Pages under medical alarms.

Elders can also avail themselves of social visits from volunteers, or enrol in an intergenerational program that links seniors with young people who, for a small fee, will be willing to help out with chores such as grass cutting and window cleaning. Alternatively, grandchildren can be a big help to their grandparents with home maintenance; they can earn a little pocket money this way, while strengthening their relationship with their grandparents. Peter's cutting the grass is a good example of this.

For elders who crave outside contact, there are centres for the elderly across the country that offer a variety of recreational programs, social outings, cultural and educational activities, and often meals. There are also senior citizens' clubs that offer similar social, educational, and recreational opportunities. Check your Yellow Pages under 'Senior Citizen Centres' for more information. See also the appendix to this book.

Services for Seniors Needing Home Health Care

But what if more is needed? What if the elder is disabled, or frail, or has suffered a stroke that limits his or her mobility? Also, what happens when a hospitalized elder such as Rebecca's mother comes home and needs extra care for a time? Most elderly don't need the round-the-clock care that hospitals provide. With help from professional services such as home care, nursing, and homemaking, many of these elderly can stay home.

For those who have been assessed as needing more than just the basic necessities, home health care is the next step. Home care programs are available throughout the country for those who need some personal care and health care. These programs offer homemaking services and varying amounts of nursing care, from one to four hours a day. Home care programs revolve around acute short-term care, such as is needed when a person comes home from hospital with an injury that will heal, as well as chronic, long-term care for elders who, with some daily health care, can remain in their own homes. The same programs also offer terminal care for dying elders. In some provinces the elder's doctor must apply for home care; the elder is then assigned to a case manager, who works with the family and assesses the elder's needs. In other provinces the elder can ask for the care directly. Care may include any combination of nursing, physiotherapy, speech and occupational therapy, and so on. Homemakers may come in daily and attend to such basics as housekeeping, meals, washing, dressing, grooming, laundry and cooking.

Many of Canada's home care programs are funded by government but also rely heavily on volunteers and donations. Sometimes there is a nominal fee, but usually basic services are free to eligible seniors, or offered on a sliding scale according to economic need. Costs vary depending on where the elder lives and on his or her needs. Clients must contact these agencies directly to obtain service, and especially in rural areas may have to contact several to get the full range of services required. Clients may buy services beyond those funded by home care or Medicare, such as twenty-four-hour care, if they have the financial means. The Victorian Order of Nurses, the Canadian Red Cross, Meals on Wheels, the YWCA, Extendicare Canada, and the Canadian Home Care Association (see appendix) are but a few of the organizations that can help you, or put you in contact with those who can. In most urban areas, umbrella groups exist that can co-ordinate care as well as provide counselling and housing information. Look in your Yellow Pages for services in your area, or check with your local library, or community or seniors' centre.

Other services may be available, free of charge if warranted, such as nutritional counselling for elders who are not eating properly or who have an illness that requires a special diet. Special equipment such as walkers, IVs, beds, and other devices are also available. Many service clubs and community groups provide needed equipment and services to elders on a volunteer basis.

Some elders with the financial means may prefer a live-in housekeeper who is paid a set fee, which depending on the needs of the elder can range from free room and board in exchange for some services, to substantial fees. Some private insurance policies will cover nursing care at home, so it makes sense to check.

Some communities have a match-and-share service that matches elderly people with experienced persons, who take them into their own homes and care for them. Some elders make use of match-and-share programs that allow them to take in a compatible lodger. In such programs those involved establish their own space but also share common space. The arrangement may include an exchange of services to the elder owner, such as shopping in exchange for a reduced rent. This arrangement offers companionship and security and allows the elder to stay at home.

Young adults who are living at home and have time on their hands can help their grandparents. Grandchildren sometimes move in with their grandparents, especially if the grandparents live in another city and the grandchild is attending university there. They may get free room and board in exchange for helping out with shopping, meals, and other light chores. Many grandparents help their grandchildren materially by providing money, a place to live, and/or a car; the grandchildren can reciprocate if the grandparents one day need help of their own.

Locating Services

Where does one find out about home health care services? It depends on the services needed. Most people contact their doctor, the local public-health department, or the nearest hospital, or they check the Yellow Pages, when more comprehensive services are required. Universities often have family care centres or schools of social work that will know where to refer you for further information. You can also call your minister or rabbi, or check community boards and local papers, or ask friends and co-workers.

Most services for elders are arranged by professionals, especially the more complicated services such as therapy, day care, home help with personal care, and the providing of medical equipment and supplies. More straightforward services such as home-delivered meals, minor chores, light housekeeping, and transportation are generally arranged by the elder or a souciaire.

What Happens If Elders Refuse Care?

What if an elder refuses any outside care and insists on a son or daughter doing it all? Rebecca's father was reluctant to accept strangers into his home but readily understood when Rebecca broached the subject. Other old people may not be so malleable. No son or daughter will allow parents to eat poorly or become ill because of a refusal to accept outside help. Stubborn, self-centred elderly parents can place a huge burden on their children. Often such a lack of judgment in an elderly person is a symptom of an illness. The souciaire may well need counselling to learn how to deal with stubborn or intimidating parents. You must learn to communicate your own needs so that the elder realizes what the choice is: outside help, or angry, resentful help from a souciaire who is burning out. Talk to your family doctor and find out what sort of counselling is available to suit your elder's needs. Most elderly can have the problems explained to them, and come to see that their needs cannot be met at the exclusive sacrifice of their children, and that they must be flexible and allow outside help. Legal remedies, such as obtaining power of attorney, are a last resort, to be used only if an elder becomes unable to make rational decisions.

*   *   *

Things got easier after Dad arranged for Meals on Wheels, and we helped him hire a housekeeper once a week for two hours. We called and dropped in on him two or three times a week, and it was no longer a constant worry for us all. Until one day I called five times and got no answer at all, on an afternoon when, I knew, Molly the cleaning woman should have been there.

I drove over after work. When I knocked on his door I got no response. I fumbled for my key, my worry edging toward panic. I raced into the living room calling his name, and checked in all the rooms before heading to the bedroom, but he wasn't there either. I tore outside into the yard and there he was. He was crumpled beside his walker, and the wooden flower box he had been trying to hang was in splinters around him. I stopped in my tracks as our eyes met.

'What took you so long?' he asked, forcing a smile.

I tried to hide my alarm and fear, but from the look in his eyes I wasn't succeeding. I didn't know what to do.

'I'm OK, Becca,' he said gently. 'I just hadn't the strength to pull myself up after I fell and the neigbours don't seem to be around to hear me calling.' He paused and then smiled. 'Whoever said old age isn't for sissies was very wise.'

He didn't *look* OK. His face was pale and pasty and he was breathing hard. I was afraid he was having a heart attack and I had no idea what to do to help him. I was scared to move him in case he had hurt his back, so I raced into the house and called an ambulance and then came back and covered him up with blankets. To hide my fear, I said–

'Dad, what happened to the housekeeper? What happened to Molly?'

'I fired her yesterday,' he said. 'Meals on Wheels too.'

When I didn't say anything, he looked at me reproachfully.

'Becca, there were just too many strange people wandering around my house.'

'Why didn't you tell someone, Dad?'

'I did. I called you at home last night and told you specifically.'

I felt a chill creep through me. He thought he'd phoned me, and maybe he had in his mind, but he hadn't *actually* phoned me. He couldn't have – I'd been out of town at a library convention, and he knew that. He had agreed to have Peter over for a game of chess, and Peter had told me they'd had a grand time and that he still couldn't beat his grandfather. Then again, perhaps he'd called one of my siblings and had just forgotten which one – not a huge lapse in memory after all. We all do it. I tried not to shiver as I realized I might not have phoned him at all today if I hadn't had something I wanted to ask his advice about. He could have lain there for many more hours believing we knew he no longer had Molly or Meals on Wheels, and waiting for someone to come and check on him.

As the ambulance arrived and we went to the hospital and the doctors pronounced him well, though bruised, I made up my mind to invite him to come and live with us, at least until Mum came home. I couldn't bear the thought of having him fall again and waiting for hours for someone to come. Every time I phoned and didn't get him, I'd worry he'd fallen again. Besides, if he moved in with us he'd eat well and I wouldn't have to worry that he'd forget to turn off the stove. But when I broached the subject as I was driving him home from the hospital, he stared at me in amazement.

'But I don't *want* to move in with you, Rebecca. I have all my friends here and my privacy and I'm doing just fine. I can get another housekeeper.

'But it's for the best, Dad, at least until Mum gets well.'

'Who says so? You or me?'

'I can't do it all. I can't be there for you all the time. Neither can Matthew or Heather or Sharon and ... and ...' I stumbled for the right words.

He slowly shook his head. In exasperation I said–

'Dad, I'm not spending enough time with my children, my husband. I love you but I love them too and they need me as well. If you come and stay with us for a while it'll be easier for all of us. It'll just be temporary until Mum comes back.'

'And what if she doesn't, Becca? '

'Don't talk like that, Dad. She'll be back.'

'Why is it only the old can talk about death, Becca? She may not come back, you know, and if she does she can't keep caring for me. You pointed that out to me yourself. It's why I agreed to Molly. Things are going to have to change – your mother and I both know that. But it doesn't mean we can't remain independent and stay living here as long as we can.'

We watched each other in silence.

'It'll only be temporary, Dad, and besides, Mum is worried you're not eating properly.'

He smiled.

'Temporary has a habit of becoming permanent, Rebecca.'

But I didn't listen. I was too busy planning how to persuade David to move back into the basement so Dad could have Danielle's ground-floor room.

*   *   *

Should Your Parents Live with You?

Rebecca did not give a lot of thought to asking her father to move in temporarily, and did not talk it over with her family or her parents in more than a superficial way. In short, she panicked, and decisions made in a panic often turn out to be poor ones. What should she have done instead?

How do you decide to invite your parents to live with you, assuming you have the room? Should you? Experts suggest that you should not unless you have no recourse. Most parents do not live with their children, and most do not want to, and this should ease any misplaced guilt you may be harbouring about not inviting your parents home. Older people prefer to be independent, just as we all do. They want to continue to live on their own. They see moving in with their children as the loss of independence it is, and many are also afraid of being a burden.

A 1996 Angus Reid survey found that only 6 per cent of Canadians say they have elderly parents living with them. As education and income increase, the likelihood that parents are living with their adult children decreases. The same survey found that one in four Canadians expect their elders to move in with them, but expectations are higher among younger Canadians 18 to 34 than older Canadians.

So what are your responsibilities to your elders? Many of you will one day have to accept that even with help you won't be able to care for your parents in their own home. How long should caregiving go on? When is enough enough? Unfortunately, standard answers to these questions don't exist because of vast individual differences among families, and because none of us can be completely objective. Rebecca is sure the move will be temporary, and that when her mother returns home all will be normal again. But will it be? She should be aware, as her father said, that temporary can turn permanent. The decision to invite a parent to move in should take in all scenarios, and you and your elders and the other souciaires should discuss the decision, and agree on all apsects of it, before any move is made.

Don't Act Prematurely

It is critical to listen to your elders and not push them into something that may be less appealing than their present situation. If you move your mother from her home into yours, or into a home nearby, it could backfire. Before pushing for such a change, you must know all the facts and understand the potential impact. Consider what your parents are leaving behind. Moving them away from their social network and in with you may help ease your worries about them getting hurt physically or not eating well, but it may also bring about emotional problems such as depression as they struggle to replace what they have lost. Make sure you are not making the decision for your own peace of mind. Make sure you consider *their* point of view, and don't force them into anything prematurely. It is hard to make decisions about someone else's life, and almost certainly you will second-guess yourself. Make sure you know what they want by discussing it with them, just as you would want them to discuss with you any plans they might have for you.

Questions to Ask before Your Elders Move In

Before inviting your elders to live with you, realize that having them under your roof will probably be much more stressful than taking care of them in their own home. After all, everyone is going to be giving up some autonomy. You need to evaluate carefully how it will affect everyone, and have a family discussion that covers the following questions:

- Who's going to do the housework, cooking, personal care, and so on? Also, what will be the role of the siblings? When an elder moves in, siblings often do less, as they perceive that help is not as necessary as it was before.
- How will it affect your work? Will you have to cut back or quit your job? Can you afford to do that?
- If finances are an issue, what will the arrangements be? Who will pay for what?

- What rules will be needed for privacy, and for entertainment, and for mediating among the three generations?
- If the primary souciaire must go away and the elders cannot be left alone, who will take over, and what will the arrangements be?
- What sort of medical problems do your elders have, and how much do you know about it?

Understanding the Health Problems of the Elderly

Souciaires need to understand the health problems of their elders so that they can assess their own ability to provide care and to meet their elders' needs. Both souciaires and elders need to be educated in the symptoms of illness and how to recognize and even prevent them. They must also learn how illnesses progress, and how they may affect the elderly in the long term. Many souciaires complain that they lack the information about elders' health that would enable them to evaluate changing behaviour. Examples: How does one tell the difference between Alzheimer's and normal memory loss? between an impending heart attack and indigestion? Another example: Most people don't die from stroke; rather, they become disabled, and the older the person the greater the risk of stroke. A souciaire who knows how to recognize the symptoms of stroke can ensure that the elder receives anticoagulants early, which will reduce the chances of disability. Both souciaires and elders need to learn about the psychological, physical, and social aspects of aging. Especially after eighty-five, the elderly are likely to face serious medical problems such as these: arthritis, rheumatism, cardiovascular problems, bowel and urinary problems, respiratory problems, stomach and digestion problems, stroke and the effects of stroke, dizziness, hearing loss, high blood pressure, loss of vision, depression, Alzheimer's, cancer, and diabetes. The elderly face many other losses as well – of status, prestige, power, friends, income, pets, and family. Younger people can bounce back from illness, but the frail do not usually have the opportunity. This can lead to depression, fear, and inactivity; as losses accumualte, dependence on others grows.

Education about the health problems of the elderly can help people like Rebecca avoid or reduce many difficulties associated with caregiving. Also, it can give both souciaires and elders the confidence to make wise decisions. Groups such as Alzheimer Society of Canada, the Arthritis Society, the Canadian Cancer Society, the Osteoporosis Society of Canada, the Heart and Stroke Foundation, and the Suicide Information and Education Centre can provide specific information; such groups as the American Association of Retired Persons and Seniorsnet on the Internet can provide both general and specific information on many topics (see Resources in the appendix). Also, don't overlook your local library.

Plan Ahead

Souciaires should realize that if they invite their elders to live with them, they should have a plan regarding who will care for them when the souciaire needs a break, if the elders' health has deteriorated to the point where a geat deal of supervision is needed. Respite care and similar programs are not substitutes for getting others in the family to share the load. If for whatever reason there is no one else to help, check to see if there is any elder day care in your area where elders can go for a few hours a day or a week. Also, find out if respite care is available in your area. Many nursing homes will care for elderly for a limited time – usually a week or two while the primary souciaire takes a holiday. Fees will depend on need and on the ability of the elder to pay.

Adult day programs are available at many hospitals and community centres, and at some residential facilities; these can help elders who have speech, memory, and mobility difficulties. The Victorian Order of Nurses offers adult day care for about $13 a day, which includes two snacks, transportation, and counselling. Some service groups also offer respite care or day care companion services, as well as parent sitting in the souciaire's home. Some of these organizations charge nothing, or a minimal fee. Finally, in many regions there are co-ordinating services that for a fee will help you find respite, day care, and other services. For more information on all of the above, see the Resources section on the appendix.

*   *   *

Dad reluctantly moved in with us two days later, and ten days after that Mum arrived in a weakened state from her stroke. That's when things began to disintegrate. Our small house grew smaller still as Mum moved into Danielle's room with Dad.

David and I were waiting in line for the bathroom and I could feel his anger simmering. Suddenly he blurted out–

'Mum, you said it was going to be temporary, that when Gramps and Grandma move out I can move into Danielle's room. So how long is temporary?'

How long indeed, I thought.

'Yeah,' piped up Peter, who had joined us in the line. 'How long do I have to put up with David trying to bribe me to swap rooms with him?'

I gave David a dirty look, but he just shrugged sheepishly and looked away.

'I can't even play music in my room after school because one or the other of them is having a nap, but it's the middle of the day, Mum, and you always said it's OK as long as it's not past eleven at night.'

'And then they stay up watching TV till all hours and it's up loud so they can hear,' said David, adding his two cents. 'And they're usually watching some weird educational shows when my friends and I want to watch soccer or tennis.'

'Guys,' I said, 'look, I know, it's not easy, but we have to learn to compromise.' I was wishing *they*'d watch some of those weird educational shows for a change.

'But we feel like *we*'re doing all the compromising – no music, no loud noise, no staying out too late or we'll wake everyone, no hogging the bathroom, and no complaining about others hogging the bathroom.' Peter looked pointedly at the closed door.

'Guys ...' I said, in what must have been my lecturing voice.

'We know, we know. Compromise, compromise.'

I smiled. Things weren't so bad most of the time. Nothing was one-sided. The kids could be loud and messy and inconsiderate but Mum and Dad were quite set in their own ways. I knew they missed their independence. There was bound to be friction. There were other things, too, that just seemed to grind me down, nibbling away at my sanity, including our glaring lack of privacy from our children and our parents and my frustration at never being able to mediate arguments very well.

*   *   *

Power Struggles

Three generations living under one roof can mean three different ways of looking at life, and privacy issues can become even more loaded with three generations than when two generations are living together. Your children may want loud music and total freedom to leave their rooms messy or tidy. You may be ready to tolerate some loud music and messy rooms but put your foot down when guests come. Your parents may be unable to tolerate any loud music and may complain about your lack of control over your own children. They may criticize how you have raised them and want to impose their own values on you and your children. They may not be flexible enough to understand that a 10 p.m. curfew for your sixteen-year-old is unrealistic in today's world. Just like your children, your elders must learn to live in your household under your rules; but there must also be some flexibility and respect for all or the situation will deteriorate. Compromise and communication are paramount.

Your parents may find it difficult not to treat you like a child in your own home, and may complain that you stay out too late, or want to know where you have been and everything you have done. Power struggles can become pronounced once your elders move in with you and you must be aware that their loss of independence may be hard for them to accept. It is important that they retain as much control over their lives as possible without adversely affecting others. In some unfortunate situations, the elder holds power over the souciaire to such an extreme that the souciaire never goes away and never gets a vacation because the parent is so demanding, needs so much, and refuses to let anyone else help. If this situation describes you, you need to seek counselling in order to break the cycle, because it is this kind of care that burns souciaires out, and a burned out souciaire is of no help to anyone. Talk to your family doctor and see what help is available.

Grandparent/Grandchild Conflicts

Your children may find it difficult to get along with their grandparents in such closed quarters, where the impatience of youth and the stubbornness of age meet headlong. When the relationship between grandparents and grandchildren is poor, this can place enormous stress on the souciaire, who must mediate. If a grandmother is annoyed that her grandchildren don't go to church, or hates the clothes they wear or the late hours they keep, the souciaire may have to translate her feelings to the grandchildren so that they understand, and then interpret the grandchildren's feelings to the grandmother so that she understands. Usually the souciaire is the peacekeeper and needs to keep on top of things at all times to maintain the peace. If in this combined role you are having problems keeping the peace, admit it. Face it head on. Get the facts. Get all the generations together and talk it out and come to a solution you can all live with. Family meetings or councils are a good way to find out what everyone is thinking. Whoever leads the council must try and anticipate all the difficulties that may arise and defuse them as much as possible before the meeting actually takes place. The point is to get everyone to walk a mile in each others' shoes.

Suggestions for Coping

Be considerate, be a good listener, be positive, establish priorities, set limits, develop good support systems, and educate your children about their responsibilities to their grandparents, to you and to themselves. Be supportive, and encourage all to be independent, and then ask for help when you need it. Make things as easy as you can for yourself. Hire someone to do your housecleaning if you can afford it, or better yet, get the whole family to chip in. If you have trouble with kids not making their beds, buy duvets; if dishes continually pile up, hide your extra dishes and leave out only enough for each family member. Do the same for towels, making sure everyone has a special design or colour. Buy clothes that don't need any ironing, have your kids make their own school lunches, eat dinner together and take turns making it. Make sure things don't all fall on your shoulders, and educate your family in the fine art of caring. The family as a whole should take responsibility. Living together as a group requires every member to be thoughtful, to treat all others in an honest, open manner, and to take on a fair share of the work.

Three-generational living can be a wonderful experience, with all three generations learning from each other and grandparents and grandchildren developing a special relationship. Don't hesitate to consult the elderly on family issues or on how to raise a child. Elders can act as role models on how to raise kids and how to age gracefully and with wisdom. We can learn much from our elders.

Family Counselling

But what happens if none of this seems to work? The tension remains, and the quarrelling increases. You may need family counselling if your family is having difficulty interacting and solving problems in a positive manner. It is important to recognize this need and not hide from it, since caregiving can permanently affect your health if you don't look after yourself. Social workers can provide help for families in communication skills such as listening, expressing feelings, and empathizing; they can also suggest strategies for getting all family members to help. Your family doctor can help get the ball rolling (or, see Resources in the appendix for more information). Communicating across the generations or with cognitively impaired elders may require new skills, and social workers can help you develop those skills. You can learn how to manage stress, improve your problem-solving skills, and deal with family issues, conflict, and guilt. If you can't get your men folk to help, there is counselling to help you get the men in your life more involved.

Some souciaires are uncomfortable about seeking counselling or joining support groups; if so, they can take advantage of information and lectures on a wide range of topics, ranging from how to care for the cognitively impaired to dealing with guilt and anger. Although this book cannot delve into the special needs of souciaires caring for cognitively impaired elders, there are many support groups and information resources available. Social workers and senior citizens' groups can tell you where they are (see Resources in the appendix).

*   *   *

In the quiet of the library the phone always rang piercingly loud, especially when it was for me. And it had been for me a lot lately as I tried to help organize medical care for Mum until she recovered and she and Dad could move home.

Ginette, my boss, handed the receiver over to me with a pointed look that said, in no uncertain terms, *no private stuff on library time.* Over the months, I'd had to fake being sick in order to get the time off to do things for my parents, send money to Danielle, or leave early to watch Peter's drama production, since my boss had warned me about being late for work too often. What else could I have done?

Today it was the local community centre saying they had to cancel transportation to next week's day program on using the Internet, and that I or one of my family would have to drive Dad there. I hung up and ran my hands distractedly through my hair and then jumped as a shadow fell over my desk.

My boss was standing over me, fiddling with a pencil and looking embarrassed. 'Look,' she said, 'I couldn't help but overhear that conversation and it sounded like private stuff. You've been doing too much of that, Rebecca. Do it on your own time, not the library's.'

Listening to her, I suddenly felt like laughing – one huge, hysterical, never-ending guffaw. How could I make someone understand my predicament who had never experienced it herself? How was I supposed to do this on my own time when most of the people I needed to deal with had left work by the time I got home or were on their lunch hour when I was? I almost let her walk away from me without saying anything, but then something snapped inside me.

'Do you have parents, Ginette?' I asked.

She turned and eyed me curiously. 'What's that got to do with it?'

'Everything,' I said. 'I'm holding down a full-time job and trying to care for my parents and my children at the same time.'

'Why can't your parents care for themselves?' she asked, her voice clipped and cold.

'Because they're getting old.'

'So am I,' she said glibly. I figured with that answer she was a lost cause. At fifty-five she was not exactly old, but I gave it one more try.

'I mean *old* in the sense that you find it difficult to button up your pants in the morning, and impossible to open a can of soup for lunch because your hands are riddled with arthritis, and you can't read simple instructions on pill bottles because your eyes aren't as good as they used to be. I'm talking about being unable to read a book because your concentration wanders or because you forget what came before. I'm talking about old as in disabled from a stroke, and you can't get your tongue around once familiar words so that the wrong words come out, but in your head you know what you want to say. I'm talking about the desperate need for help from family but the reluctance to lose your independence, the fear of having a stroke or another heart attack, the inability to drive anymore because of your disabilities and the need to have someone take you to all your medical appointments and any and all social events because you can't get there in your walker or your wheelchair.'

When I'd finished, there was dead silence, and I saw that many of my co-workers had gathered around. I let the silence linger a while longer and then let the anger and resentment keep pouring out –

'There are lots of us out there trying desperately to help our elderly parents and keep our jobs at the same time, without feeling we're being discriminated against. We get really good at deception, calling in sick when actually we need to take our parents to medical tests, or arriving late and pleading a flat tire when we've just had to spend more time than usual helping our parents get dressed and fed. Or sneaking in all sorts of calls during working hours, like criminals, to try and arrange for care and management of our parents when other plans have fallen through.'

I paused, searching for the right words to try and make her understand.

'We can't ignore them,' I said, 'just like we can't ignore our kids when they get sick. The library has a day care centre, so it's recognized the problems of parents with young children. But what about parents whose *parents* need them? We could do with some understanding.'

Many of my co-workers were silently nodding. That bolstered my confidence a bit, and on I went –

'We could do with flexible hours. Why can't we be an hour late and make up the time after work? Or take a longer lunch so that we can get our parents to the dentist or the doctor during office hours? We need help so that we can do our jobs without the distractions of having to juggle company time with private time.'

I stopped then, and wondered whether I had gone too far. It was such a public venue I felt I could have written my resignation letter then and there, but life can surprising. I had hit a nerve somewhere, and the emotions that played across her face left no doubt that she actually knew what I was talking about. I wondered then about her own parents. Were they still alive?

She simply asked, 'Why didn't you tell me all this before?' And then she looked around at the rest of the employees, many my age and older, and said –

'How many of you are in the same boat?'

I was surprised to see several hands go up. She turned back to me and said –

'Get some information on what other companies are doing to handle this and let me know. We'll take it from there, but I'm not promising anything.'

She turned to go, but then called back over her shoulder –

'And Rebecca? Make sure you find out about how to take care of yourself as well as your parents.'

*   *   *

Employers Need a Wake-up Call

If you are one of the really lucky ones, like Rebecca, you may be able to get resources and information from your employer to help you with your caregiving.

Most employers are still in the Stone Age when it comes to elder care, and the Dark Ages when it comes to child care; this is changing, however, as employers begin to realize that these issues may be affecting their bottom line. They are starting to look at losses linked to elder and child care such as arise from absenteeism, tardiness, missed meetings, increased use of sick days, poor performance, increased turnover of employees, and reduced productivity. All of these translate into lower profits. Unfortunately, many employers are not supportive of souciaires who work; or, like Ginette, they are simply unaware of the problem.

Employers Take Note When Their Bottom Line Is Affected

Employer interest has been a long time coming, especially when you consider that business has for years been a net beneficiary of the unpaid care that souciaires give. The contribution that souciaires make to society has always been ignored in the profit base. But businesses are beginning to take note that child and elder care issues affect them – and none too soon, as it has been estimated that in the next decade 60 per cent of growth in the labour force will be women 35 to 54 (1, 2). Estimates of how many employees care for their elders vary according to the definition of care; percentages range from 16 to 23 per cent of Canadian workers. One study of 10,000 souciaires found that 38 per cent of employees had been providing care for more than five years, and 11 per cent for more than ten (3).

Employer Initiatives Are Rare

Caring for the elderly is set to become a critical workplace issue. More and more businesses are discovering that helping employees find ways to care for the young and the old improve both competitiveness and job performance. Some companies have innovative programs that provide information and counselling for employees who must deal with elder care and stress. Some firms hold seminars on what is available in the community, and some publish booklets on, for example, how to choose a nursing home. Some have contracts with consulting firms that help employees manage care even at a distance. Managing the care of elders can be time consuming, from negotiating and making arrangements, to checking and hiring helpers, and employers need to address this by being as flexible as the job allows. Some offer flexible working hours so that employees can help elders get dressed or drive them to appointments. If a company does not permit employees to use sick days to help elders, the employees will do it anyway and hide it. If possible, the company should let employees come in late and work late, or job share.

More firms are giving unpaid leave to employees with family problems, and some now grant every employee a number of family care days per year. Some have special insurance to help employees pay for care. Others permit employees to take leave if an elder needs help, or to work a twelve-hour weekend day for a full week's pay and full benefits. Some pay out a subsidy indexed to a paycheque for eldercare and child care.

Other initiatives taken by the rare employer include support groups, counselling, education, and training. Some employers have set up information and educational seminars over lunch hour and offer guidance on how to find needed services. Many employees need only partial care for their parents but often cannot find it. Employees appreciate these employee assistance programs. The easy availability of options provides a safety net for employees; just knowing they are there if needed reduces stress and increases productivity and morale. It is, however, imperative for employees to feel confident that they are not jeopardizing their careers by using the offered benefits. Workers must also guard themselves against those employers who view employees who care for elders as a liability; this attitude can lead to hiring practices that discourage hiring of souciaires – something that affects women in all fields of employment.

The search for innovative solutions to the problems of caring for elders has only just begun. There are more and more elders in our society, and there will be fewer and fewer souciaires to care for them, so a great deal remains to be done if the needs of both groups are to be met. The services discussed in this chapter are all too often difficult to find, or poorly funded, or simply not available in some communities. Clearly, we in this society are not meeting existing needs, nor are we preparing to meet the increased needs projected for the future.

The Economic Value of Unpaid Caregiving

Unfortunately, the future doesn't look particularly bright: the new leaner, meaner era of tightened budgets, hospital closures, early discharges, and day surgery means more reliance than ever on community support – or, to be accurate, on women's voluntary caring. It is cheaper to have someone cared for voluntarily at home than it is to care for a patient twenty-four hours a day in a hospital; often it is also the best thing for the patient. Unfortunately, this shift in focus to community and home care – a euphemism for women's caring – relies in large part on the self-sacrifice of volunteer souciaires at a time when more and more of them are now working full time. Souciaires are expected to donate services that help underpin our national economy, yet their caring work is grossly undervalued. Governments are quick to espouse the benefits of getting souciaires to take on the extra work, but they don't take into account the emotional and financial toll. Governments still have trouble understanding that after variables such as emotional and physical toll and lost days at work are factored in, their policies are not as cost effective as they think. Many businesses are beginning to realize this. It is time for governments to do the same, and begin to put the money they are saving through hospital restructuring back into much-needed community services. Souciaires can no longer remain invisible. Their work must be included on the balance sheet of the nation (4).

The economic value of caring must be acknowledged through the provision of supportive work policies and services. The underlying assumption that it is women who do the caring must be challenged by all Canadians. Community projects aimed at supporting souciaires must address gender inequities from the start, if they are to work. Canadians must begin to challenge the long-held assumptions about who should care and how care should be provided. We must ensure that both men and women do their share of caring for both the young and the old. Boys and girls need to be taught at an early age that the job of caring is not dependent on gender.

Unfortunately, many women still think they're alone and that they must do it all. They are not asking where their husbands, fathers, and sons are – they still believe it's up to them. Canadians cannot take such care for granted anymore, and must fund the support systems, counselling, and education needed to spread the load. The alternative is massive souciaire burnout, and all the social and financial costs that go with it.

Suggestions for Souciaires

Souciaires should take advantage of local resources to help lighten their load – and this includes looking after their own needs. Unfortunately, few souciaires report using any services geared to them, although many take advantage of programs designed to help the elderly (and, more indirectly, themselves) (5). Many souciaires feel they don't need any help for themselves; others are reluctant to ask for help because they want to be 100 per cent supportive and feel that asking for help would be an admission of failure. Many souciaires end up neglecting themselves in the rush to help others. Don't do it. If you neglect yourself you will eventually short-change everyone. Here is some good advice:

- Relax, and find some things that you really enjoy doing. Play squash with a friend, take up skydiving, develop new hobbies, go back to school or take correspondence courses, take a day off work and use it just for yourself and no one else.
- Make time to read all those books you've been wanting to read.
- Develop new friends, and touch base with old ones.
- Take pride in your job.
- Get regular exercise.
- Eat well – make time for three square meals a day.
- Use any services that are available to you to help make your life easier, and lobby for more services.

- Get a paying job, and take pride in your work.
- Volunteer for things other than caregiving.
- Learn to manage relations and emotions.
- If you smoke, give it up.
- Don't hold everything in. If you are angry, frustrated, or hurt, or feel guilty or betrayed, talk to friends or to your spouse about your feelings. You are in charge, and you must maintain a good quality of life.
- Build a support system of friends and family, or attend local support groups. If you need more, seek counselling with professional social workers or psychologists, who can act as objective observers and offer new perspectives on your problems. Get help to deal with any feelings of guilt and anger over your role as primary souciaire. Confront any guilt over feeling that caring for your elders is a burden, and realize that all souciaires feel that way at times.
- Stretch yourself, and don't stop socializing.
- Make sure your expectations are realistic.
- Make time for yourself and your spouse.
- Often the easiest thing to do is cut out things you like in order to make time for the needs of others. Be aware of how easy and insidious this can be, and don't make it a habit. No matter how much is demanded of you, you must take time for yourself.

CHAPTER SEVEN

Planning for the Future

I'd had to stay later at work than I had anticipated, to organize a lunchtime seminar on caregiving for the young and the elderly, and I didn't make it home until six. I was hoping to arrive to the smell of dinner cooking, but when I let myself into the kitchen there was nothing except a note saying they had all gone to pick up Mum from rehab and were then going to catch the end of Peter's baseball game before coming home for dinner. I sighed and took some burgers out of the freezer, then dumped some potatoes in the oven and went to take a nice long shower.

Even little things were beginning to loom large. I eyed the bathroom in distaste, no single thing I saw worth a second look but all things together weighing heavy. There were wet towels on the floor, the lid on the toothpaste tube was off, Dad's shaving stuff was scattered around the sink, the lid was up on the toilet seat, and a new roll of toilet paper had been taken out but not put in the roller. There was a ring around the bathtub, and a brandy snifter was still sitting on the edge of the tub. (I'd been watching it there for several weeks, hoping its owner would take it down to the kitchen.) Someone had taken all the clean laundry and thrown it into the dirty-laundry hamper. Mum's creams and potions were struggling with the soap and toothpaste for space on the shelf, and she'd hidden my favourite dress, which she hated, at the bottom of the linen closet. And earlier I'd found chip bags in David's room, mouldy bread in Peter's, and cookies in Dad's. Things just weren't working out.

I couldn't get through to Mum and Dad that the kids needed to be able to listen to some music, and I couldn't make the kids see that Mum and Dad were entitled to watch educational TV instead of having to give it up for a soccer match. My siblings had all but abandoned me, thinking I was just fine now that I didn't have to travel to help Mum and Dad. I was beginning to think that despite the good times, I hadn't thought through my invitation very carefully – not with David, and not with my parents – and that Dad had been wiser than I in realizing what might be in store for all of us. Now that they were living with us, how was I supposed to ask them all to leave? I wished we'd discussed all this before Dad had moved in during the winter. He should have insisted, since he seemed to know what I was getting myself into.

I walked down the hall with the dirty laundry past the door to the living room and was startled to find Dad in there listening to music with some earphones on and drumming his foot to an unheard beat. He jumped when he saw me but took off the earphones and said –

'I found Peter and David some earphones at the garage sale next door so you won't have to listen to that loud and awful music of theirs.'

I smiled at his inability to admit that he had really bought them for himself, so he wouldn't have to listen to *their* music. As if he'd read my thoughts, he smiled and said –

'I didn't buy them for myself, you know.'

When he saw my sceptical look, he added –

'Oh, don't get me wrong. I would have, but you'll be needing them more than we will.'

I caught a note of excitement in his voice and asked cautiously –

'What do you mean?'

'To be blunt, Rebecca, this waiting in line for the bathroom is just too much in my old age. We're moving out.'

Every emotion I could think of galloped through my head, from joy to guilt to fear to anger to amazement to resentment, and I blurted out the first thing that came into my head.

'We can build another bathroom.' I couldn't believe I'd said that. Neither could Dad, judging by the comical look of astonishment on his face. Both of us knew we couldn't afford to build a second bathroom.

'Really, Rebecca – I was just using the bathroom as an example. Unless you've been tuning out these past weeks, you must know that we're getting in each other's hair.' He chuckled and added, 'And that, theoretically, should be getting harder to do, not easier.'

When I looked at him in puzzlement, he smiled.

'Considering I don't have much hair left. Seriously, Rebecca, we're used to our own lifestyle. It's not working. It's too noisy for us, too quiet for your kids, and there's not enough privacy. We've been fighting like cats and dogs. We want to go home, Becca.'

I felt immense relief – I'd been afraid they would grow accustomed to being with us and that I wouldn't know how to broach the subject to them. But then I felt worried and fearful that all the old problems of caring for them in their own home would resurface, in spades.

'But you won't be able to manage at home and I can't give you the kind of care you need,' I said, feeling the guilt begin to stir.

'We'll look into services. We can get Meals on Wheels and hire Molly back again,' said my father as if he had forgotten we'd tried that before.

'Dad, be reasonable. That wasn't working and it won't work now. Mum won't be able to stop herself from trying to do it all and saving some money. You know that.'

We watched each other glumly as the tinny sounds of Beethoven's Ninth drifted up to me from the earphones on his lap. I reluctantly broke the silence, and as I did I felt the guilt well up in me like a live beast.

'You could try one of those neat seniors' complexes. You know, where you have your own place without any of the hassles of ownership. You wouldn't have to worry about repairs and all that stuff anymore. We could look into it, maybe find a reasonably priced place. I have some brochures,' I added lamely, feeling like an ungrateful daughter because I was unable to give them what they needed.

But Dad was shaking his head. 'It'd be nice, Rebecca, but your mother would never agree to leave her home after fifty years of living there, and I don't know if we could afford a place like that.'

'How do you know? Have you asked her?' Now exasperation and anger were mingling with my guilt.

'No,' he said, with a finality that signalled the end of the conversation.

He turned away from me then, and I went to the basement to do the laundry and wrestle with the feelings of guilt that were threatening to overwhelm me. As I was putting in a load, the rest of my family returned from Peter's baseball game. When I finally came upstairs, Mum was sitting in the kitchen telling Peter how to spice the burgers. He was just finishing as I walked in, and he grabbed a fistful of cutlery and headed into the dining room to set the table.

Mum was looking much better and had fairly good mobility on her left side, considering everything, but she was much weaker and unsteadier on her feet than before the stroke, and the prognosis was that she would never regain full mobility. She'd never walk without a cane again. I came straight to the point.

'Dad tells me you want to move home.'

'It's no reflection on you, Rebecca, but we want our own lives back again. No, Rebecca, I know what you're going to say – that we can't do it all on our own anymore. I know that. We'll hire some help. Your father says we have some money set aside for our old age.'

When I didn't reply, she added defensively –

'It didn't work with your father because he didn't have me to mediate. You know he's awful with people but I can get around all that.'

But could she, I asked myself, in her weakened state? Did she really want to?

She saw the look in my eye and said with a sigh –

'Your father really wants to go home, Rebecca. I can't let him down. He'd hate a retirement home.'

'Would he, Mum? Have you asked him?'

'No. No, I haven't.'

'Asked me what?' said my father as he shuffled into the kitchen, the rubber feet of his walker squeaking on the linoleum.

My mother eyed me for a few pointed seconds, until I suddenly remembered that I had a good book to read and scampered away, leaving them their privacy.

*   *   *

Broaching the Subject of Retirement Homes

Sooner or later many elders will move into the realm of the oldest old and will no longer be able to remain in their own home or with their children. Like Rebecca's parents they will need more care than they can receive either at home or from a souciaire, but usually they will not need enough to require a nursing home.

Many elders do not recognize when the time has come to move, and many sons and daughters find it extremely difficult to broach the subject. The easiest approach is to bring up the subject long before it is a concern and find out what plans your parents have for the various stages of their old age. Do they have a particular retirement home in mind, or are they interested in a seniors' complex where they might own or rent their own condominium? What are their feelings about a nursing home, should they ever need one? Also, have they set aside money to help pay for their old age?

If your elders are obviously past the point of being able to live alone safely, but refuse to admit it, then you will have to take action. Sometimes a subtle approach, such as leaving pamphlets about retirement homes lying around the house, may be all that's needed to get a conversation going. Or you may just have to take the bull by the horns, as Rebecca did, and raise the subject yourself. However you approach it, don't force a decision on them. For things to work smoothly, it should be their decision.

But what if they refuse to even consider any of your proposals, let alone actually move? Unless they are cognitively impaired and a clear danger to themselves, you cannot force them to move. You may have to wait until something transpires – a fall, an increasing loss of mobility – before they are even willing to discuss the topic. It is fairly easy to plan your childrens' needs; planning for elders' needs is not as easy. You don't have the same control with your parents as you do with your children. Decisions about moving are never easy to make, and any decision you make for them may be resisted.

The Stress of Moving

Ideally, your parents will come to the decision on their own and set things in motion before it becomes obvious to you and your siblings that something must be done. This makes things much easier for you (and provides a good role model when it's time to plan your own old age). However, never underestimate how difficult and stressful it is for elders to move out of the family home or apartment, which often they have lived in for decades. It can be terribly sad both for your parents and for you, especially if you were raised there. You remember all the good times you had and wonder how it will ever be the same without the old house or apartment. Remember, however, that your parents are only leaving behind four walls and a roof. Everything that really matters comes with them, and with you, for in the end it is the people who matter, not the bricks and mortar that housed them. It is the people who harbour the memories and help make new ones, regardless of where they live.

What Are the Options?

For many relatively autonomous elders, the first step is to sell the family home (or leave the apartment) and move into a smaller and easier-to-manage one-storey home, or an apartment with an elevator, that is close to or within walking distance of a grocery store and other conveniences. Those who have the financial means may opt to rent or buy a condo in a complex where the heavy maintenance for each unit, such as plumbing and electrical work, is done by a superintendent hired by the entire complex. Others may simply rent an apartment in an old house or apartment building that is convenient to grocery stores and other shops, and rely on the landlord to maintain the building.

Retirement Homes and Seniors' Complexes

Seniors' complexes for the young 'old' are becoming quite popular. These are often condominium or apartment buildings. Some include a golf course and other recreational facilities, and some may have a central building with a restaurant and health club. These complexes can be expensive.

Many elders want something a little more structured, and that provides services other than maintenance, and retirement homes often fit this bill. These are generally operated by the private sector and offer a wide variety of amenities and services. At some retirement homes elders get minimal supervision; at others, such as luxury retirement condos, elders have access to extensive services, including personal care, health facilities, and meals for a price (which varies widely).

Retirement homes are for those who no longer want the responsibility of looking after their own place but are still largely autonomous. Usually, rooms are private or semiprivate. Some have kitchen facilities if the home does not provide all meals, and some have apartment units so that elders can either cook their own meals or go to a central dining room. In most retirement homes, nursing care is not an option; but in some regions elders may be eligible for mobile services such as physiotherapy and occupational therapy.

Most retirement homes have twenty-four-hour emergency services and security systems. Some homes do all the laundry for the residents, while others only provide the machines. Some homes have extensive recreational and social facilities, and others very few. Most are privately owned. Costs are paid by the elder in full, and vary widely depending on location and the services offered.

Homes for the Aged

Homes for the aged are another possibility. Some of these are subsidized and operated by government or charities. The services available are similar to those provided by retirement homes but are not as luxurious. You may have a room in an older house with five or six rooms and a common area. Some homes will take in only the healthy aged, so you will have to move if you get ill. The cost is generally whatever you can afford.

Nursing Homes

Nursing homes are necessary only for the small proportion of elderly who are chronically ill and require at least one-and-a-half hours of nursing care each and every day, or more medical care than can be provided at home but not enough for hospitalization. Nowadays, nursing homes are considered to be for the oldest old: generally, those who are in their mid-eighties and whose mental health is deteriorating. About 80 per cent of elders in these homes suffer from depression or some other mental disorder, and some 70 per cent have behavioural problems (1).

Nursing homes are private and licensed and can be nonprofit or commercial. Usually they offer private and semiprivate rooms, as well as dorm-style rooms (three or four in a room). They provide help for personal needs such as bathing, dressing, toileting, and getting about, and also provide twenty-four-hour nursing supervision. Fees are set by the government on a per diem basis. Elders living in private and semiprivate rooms pay extra, as do elders who need a personal nurse. For those elders who have little money, the government will pay a portion of the costs, with the elder picking up the rest, which never exceeds what the elder can afford to pay.

The decision to move an elder into a nursing home is usually made by the souciaire; the elder is often incapable of making the decision and may resist vehemently or be scared and confused. Elders, because of mental disability, may be unable to reason, or understand their surroundings; in these situations souciaires often decide to bring them into their own home. This is taking on too much: caring for the disabled elderly is a full-time job that can involve many things, including dealing with babysitters, sleep-disturbances, feeding, and incontinence.

Souciaires Who Cannot Put Their Elders in Nursing Homes

Many souciaires who can afford a nursing home continue to care for disabled elders at home because they cannot cope with the guilt of placing them in an institution. This can exact a great physical, emotional, and financial toll, and strain family relations to the limit. In situations like this it is better to find a nursing home and to learn to accept that any reluctance to do so is born out of guilt and not out of the needs of those involved. One woman agonized over placing her mother, who had Alzheimer's, in a nursing home. Only after she took the step did she realize that her mother was actually happier in the home, and that she had been too slow to take on the responsibility for making the right decision. It is important to note that elders may be much happier in a nursing home, with its routine care, than in a family situation that is dangerously overstressed. Let your elder know what is going on, and be sensitive to their needs. It is normal to deny to yourself that your elders may need a nursing home, and you have to work your way through it. People, including souciaires, are afraid to lose their autonomy. They do not like to admit that they can no longer manage on their own.

Chronic Care Hospitals

For those who are too ill to be anywhere else and who require round-the-clock medical attention, chronic care hospitals are the last step. Elders must contribute to the cost of room and board after fifty days, but health care is covered by the government.

Availability of All These Services Is Not Guaranteed

Unfortunately, not all of the above options are available in every region of the country, and some of those which are available are suboptimal. In your search for the perfect place, you may want to get some help and advice from a counsellor, doctor, or social worker. Far too often, waiting lists are long, so you will have to plan well ahead to ensure that a place will be available when you need it. Don't expect to make the decision one day and find a suitable spot the next.

Many souciaires or elders who have finally decided to arrange for a retirement home, seniors' complex, home for the aged, or nursing home end up having to wait a year or more for a vacancy because they didn't plan ahead. One woman in her seventies was caring for her ninety-seven-year-old mother. When the mother turned 102, the daughter, who was close to burning out, applied to put her mother in an institution. Her mother died three years later, before a space became available. Another daughter looked at twenty-five homes trying to find a place for her mother, who had Alzheimer's. Some of the homes were terrible, and those that were nice had long waiting lists. The situation can only get worse until governments channel more funds into programs to help the elderly.

These women, and far too many like them, had no choice but to care for their elders at home, either because they couldn't afford outside care or because there were no spaces available when the need arose. Souciaires need to know that when they need help it will be there within a reasonable time. Unfortunately, this is not presently the case, and recent government initiatives have done nothing to improve the situation. In fact, it can be argued that cutbacks have had the opposite effect.

We need a huge expansion of home services. Most souciaires also have jobs, and far too many reduce their work hours or quit when they cannot find care for their elders. They cannot abandon their parents, so they have no choice. Because of emotional ties, they cannot walk away, as they could from a job. Governments need to be lobbied for more and better facilities for our elderly.

In the meantime, plan as far ahead as you can. Get your elder's name on a number of waiting lists. Keep in touch, and ask the home whether it will accept a transfer from another establishment when there is a vacancy, in case your elders get in at their second choice first. If their name comes up but it is too soon for them to move, ask the home to keep their names on the waiting list for future need.

Suggestions for Choosing the Right Facility

But how do you know which long-term facility will be best suited for your elders' needs? Figure out what you or your parents can afford, and then visit the establishments you think would be suit-

able. Talk to the other residents, and to the staff. Eat a meal there.
Look at the following things:

- *Health facilities.* Is medical care provided for nonthreatening illnesses? Is there a doctor on call? Can residents keep their own
  doctor, or must they use the on-call doctor?
- *Nursing and personal care.* Is it provided twenty-four hours?
- *Medical equipment.* What is available for the residents? For example, are wheelchairs and walkers provided?
- *Safety.* Are there handrails in the halls? Are fire exits well marked
  and easy to negotiate? Is there a sprinkler system? Are there
  emergency buttons in the rooms?
- *Physical facilities.* Are these clean and pleasant? Are the rooms
  well lit? Are the common rooms comfortable and friendly? Is
  there a library? What recreational facilities are there? What
  social events and educational programs are there? How close
  is the home to shopping centres, libraries, and other conveniences?
- *Meals.* If the home serves them, what are they like? Are they
  nutritious, and are the helpings sufficient? Is there a dietician? Is
  the dining room a place you would want to eat everyday?
- *Linen and laundry.* Does the home provide all bedding and linen
  and do all the laundry? In general terms, does the home take
  care of all the residents' basic daily needs?
- Does the home offer safekeeping?
- *Quality of life.* Do the residents seem happy? Are the staff polite,
  friendly, and respectful? Is their morale high?
- *Family involvement.* Are families involved in planning care? Are
  they consulted?
- *Administrative policies.* What are the rules concerning meals, visi-
  tors, children, alcohol, and smoking? Are residents allowed to
  smoke in their rooms? in common areas? Can residents come
  and go as they like? Some homes have strict rules, some don't.
- *Location.* Is the home close enough to family for frequent visits?
- *Service agreement.* Take this home and study it. It should tell you
  what the home will provide and what level of care can be
  expected.

- *Licence and inspections.* Check the home's licence and current inspection report, and ask if it is accredited.
- *Costs.* To avoid unpleasant surprises, get a complete breakdown of charges, including those for extras such as a private room or apartment.
- *Continuity of care.* It's not a pleasant thought, but you should know in advance where you stand if your elders get ill. If they become too ill or mentally confused to care for themselves, will they be kicked out, or can the home transfer them to a chronic care wing or a related facility? Some homes for the aged and some retirement homes will take on cognitively impaired elders, alcoholics, or hard-to-handle elders who need additional help; but many will not because they are not equipped to handle those elders whose behaviour is disruptive (2, 3).
- *Accommodation for couples.* Elderly *couples* (as opposed to singles) have complex needs, and finding space for them may be more difficult, especially if one elder is disabled and the other is more or less still autonomous. Look for a home that provides more than one level of care, and remember that two levels of care may cost more than one.

No single place is likely to be ideal. Choose the one that best suits your elders' emotional and financial needs, and include them in the decision-making process at all times.

*   *   *

I don't know what Mum and Dad said to each other in the kitchen that day, but the upshot was a series of never-ending visits to various retirement homes, some far too expensive and some depressingly awful. Finally, they chose a small unit in a seniors' complex in the suburbs. It had most of the features they wanted and could afford. They'd had to compromise on location and on the size of their future living quarters, because so many homes closer to the city had huge waiting lists and were too expensive. The payoff was that they would be facing only a short wait. They'd put their house up for sale, which was turning into an emotional roller coaster for all of us. It isn't easy saying goodbye to a house you've known for

fifty years and the packing and moving was still ahead. I was thinking about that as I spied Mum sitting in the living room one day
staring unseeing at the wall in front of her, a cup of tea untouched
on the table in front of her. When she looked up at me as I came
into the room, there was concern on her face, not the sadness I
had feared. I looked at her questioningly.

She sighed and said –

'Your father and I are really worried about Elsie, Becca.'

'Elsie?' I asked, wondering who Elsie was.

Mum looked at me in reproach.

'You took us to her husband's funeral four months ago. She's
the wife of your father's old chess partner.'

I'd taken them to many funerals in recent months. Yes, I did
remember Dad's old chess partner, Wayne, although I didn't know
his widow well.

'She's depressed and isn't coping well with living alone, and we
don't know how to help her. I mean, I don't know how I could ever
cope with life if I lost your father. I'm terrified of that, so how can I
possibly help her?'

I didn't know how to answer. Did she want me to talk to her
about her own fears of dying, which frankly scared me too? Or did
she want me to help Elsie? Either way, I felt impotent.

'How?' asked my mother again.

The old line, 'It takes time,' seemed so cold and inadequate that
I remained silent, frozen in inadequacy. A sick feeling swept over
me as I thought about losing one of my own parents and how we
would handle that, and how hard it would be to help the survivor.
My thoughts were spinning out of control when Mum brought me
back to earth.

'It's gets worse, though.'

I must have missed something she said, and I wondered what
could be worse than losing someone you love.

'Elsie let Wayne handle all their bills,' she continued, 'and the
management of all their assets – even insurance and who to phone
if the pipes burst. She has no idea where he kept their assets, if
they have any, and no one has been able to find a will.'

'Is that a problem?'

'Apparently it is. They can't settle any of the estate until it's found, and if there's no will the government will decide for her where it all goes, meaning her delinquent son could get something he doesn't deserve. Meanwhile she has no money. His assets have been frozen – I didn't know they could do that – until the powers that be decide how to divvy it all up ... and she has bills piling up like crazy, including funeral expenses, which it doesn't look as though Wayne planned for at all. She had no idea how expensive a funeral could be. Neither did I. They can run to five thousand dollars and more! She doesn't even know if she has any pension or is entitled to any of Wayne's, now he's dead. He did it all, but she says he never planned for retirement. And no one has been able to find out if there is any life insurance. It's a real mess, and on top of all this she's in deep mourning and depressed and wants nothing to do with having to figure out finances. She's still distraught over the hospital's refusal to take him off life support after the stroke. He hadn't given any such permission, but Elsie knew it was what he wanted. They'd even talked about it. And now she's facing eviction.'

I didn't know what Mum wanted me to do. I wasn't really sure I could help much, until she dropped the bombshell and it ceased being Elsie's problem and became mine as well.

'I know as much about our finances as Elsie does about hers,' she said.

I stared at her in amazement.

'You mean ...'

She nodded in embarrassment. 'Your father has done it all over the years, and I never asked and he's never discussed it. I didn't think it was important. I don't even know if we had a will, or any insurance to cover funeral expenses, or what our investments are, or even if we have any.'

I felt a vague uneasiness as I heard my mother's description: it described more than just her. I took care of all the finances in my family, while Bryan knew practically zip. For that matter, I didn't know as much as it seemed I needed to know, and that was a startlingly unpleasant revelation.

'What are you going to do?' I asked.

'I could bury my head in the sand and forget it and hope I die first. But statistics are against me on that one. I'm likely to outlive your father and face Elsie's predicament.'

She looked at me and grinned.

'So I'm going back to school, Becca. We're enrolled in a community course at the high school on planning for the future. It includes all sorts of things like investments, wills, insurance, saving and planning for retirement or the kids' education, budgeting, living wills, power of attorney, and even Internet resources on the subject and how to access them. It even includes an optional side-kick CPR course so that if there's a heart attack in the family we'll all know what to do. Everyone thinks it's a great idea for us to all know what's going on and learn how to plan for the future. Some of us have shorter futures than others, but they say it's never too late to plan.'

My suspicions were growing with every *we* and *us* she threw in. What was she up to? I wondered.

She leaned forward and picked up her teacup and then continued –

'The pre-course material has already galvanized your father into upgrading his will and the kids into thinking about taking out RRSPs.'

She carefully placed the teacup back on the table, and smiled sweetly at me like the cat that's just eaten the pet budgie.

'Mum, what have you done?' I blurted out.

'You can thank Peter and David and Bryan,' she laughed.

'Thank them for what?' I asked uneasily.

'They've enrolled us all in the course, and it starts next Monday night.'

*   *   *

Fear of Dying

This is not the first time that Rebecca's Mum has alluded to her fears of dying, or of being left behind to live alone like Elsie. Elders may harbour many fears related to age and be unable to voice them: fear of not being able to help a loved one who is dying, fear of not doing the right thing in an emergency and then having a loved one die, fear of dying and leaving loved ones behind whose full life's story you'll never know, fear of having loved ones forget you, fear of pain and disability, fear of being left behind by loved ones and living alone in sorrow. All of us must confront our feelings and be honest about how they are affecting us. While fear of death is unpleasant, it is not uncommon; sometimes, however, this fear can become pathological to the point of paralysis. Elders who dwell too much on fears of death – their own or their loved ones' – may need counselling to help them come to terms with life's processes. They must learn how to confront their fears so that they don't descend into depression or mental paralysis, as Elsie seems to be doing. Counselling can help them achieve a healthier view of life and death and provide them with skills for coping with their fear. (Ask your family doctor for advice.) Rebecca is not keen to talk about the eventual death of her parents. This is not unusual: we all have difficulty facing the death of loved ones. But that doesn't mean we can't learn about what we can expect.

Widowhood

Perhaps no late-life change is as profound as the change from married to widowed. A person who loses a spouse loses a close and intimate friend, someone with whom to share ideas, dreams, hopes, disappointments, and day-to-day talk. Estimates are that seven out of ten women will survive their husbands, so this is largely a women's issue. However, recent research suggests that widowed men suffer more emotional pain than widowed women. Men's socialization may not have equipped them to live alone, and to cook meals for themselves and maintain a household. They may have let their wives maintain social contact with any kin, and they may suddenly find themselves isolated, and without a network of friends, especially if they are also retired and have not kept up their friendships. This may explain why more widowers than widows seek suicide (4).

The suffering one goes through at the death of a loved one has definite stages, and only time can heal the pain (though not the ache). Successful adaptation to widowhood is easier if there has been time, as in the case of a lengthy illness, to anticipate the death and come to terms with it.

Widows use their family network as the first line of support and comfort, and for economic assistance and crisis help. However, research shows that kin involvement seems to be minimal after the death of a spouse, and that the support tends to be short-term and ceremonial rather than lasting. A widow's kinship network may shrink upon widowhood, and the involvement of kin is usually limited to the children of the widow, especially daughters. Grandchildren can play a big role here, by phoning and visiting and taking their elders on outings. (5)

In time, most widows learn to live alone, and many can be very happy. However, it is important for widows to realize that they are now on their own and that friends may see them differently. They may wonder where they fit in now. They may miss the company, intimacy, and hugs that were a part of their life, and they may face days of loneliness and boredom.

They may feel a need to move out of the family home, or they may be pressured to do so. However, most people advise widows to do nothing drastic, such as selling the house or changing apartments, for at least six months to two years; they need this much time to get things into perspective. It would be sad to sell a house in grief and then six months later regret the move. To fill the void, widows should try and keep busy, and continue to do the things they had planned to do in their retirement. Some widows remarry; others buy a pet; still others take up new hobbies, return to old ones, or join new organizations and clubs. In time they can find a high degree of independence and peace.

When You Are Old – Planning Ahead

But what if you're like Elsie, who for more than fifty years has depended on her husband for everything? His death has resulted in economic disruption for her and the taking on of new and unfamiliar tasks at a time when her energy and spirits are low. Elsie's situation is not uncommon, as Rebecca has discovered: her mother is equally at sea about the family's finances, and in order to avoid Elsie's fate has set out to remedy that by taking a course on how to plan for the future.

It is never too soon to plan for your financial future. Too many widows face poverty because they did not know anything about their husband's finances. They may find that they are not entitled to the husband's pension, or that the husband saved nothing or invested any savings poorly. Husbands and wives must be aware of each other's finances – what they are worth, where they are held, and so on – even if those assets don't add up to a great deal. Women and men who do not make a point of learning all this are leaving themselves very vulnerable.

Suggestions for Planning Ahead

Some of the things you should be thinking about in terms of planning include the following:

- *Retirement.* Try to set aside enough money each year that you will be able to maintain the same standard of living in your old age. If you have a company pension plan, check to see what benefits would be due to you and to your spouse should you die. Get your bank or a certified financial advisor to tell you whether that amount of money will be enough. There are computer programs available that will run through endless scenarios for you, taking into account the impact of inflation and earned interest on any money you set aside. These programs can tell you the minimum amount you will need for your retirement. Ask your bank for more information.
- *RRSPs.* If you are self-employed with no pension, or if your pension is not going to be enough, try to contribute to a registered retirement savings plan (RRSP) every year, starting as soon as you are able. Even just $100 a year, if it earns compound interest, can grow to a tidy sum over the years. Many women's pensions are considerably lower than men's because of their work history – taking time off to have a baby, or being hired for lower-paying jobs. Remember that RRSPs are tax sheltered; in other words, in

all tax brackets the cost of your yearly contribution is less than if
you were not allowed to deduct the amount from your income.
It's never too soon to plan for your retirement, because the
money grows in value and is tax sheltered until you use it. Again,
ask for help at your bank. Elders today can take advantage of the
Canada Pension Plan and the Old Age Supplement, but there is
no guarantee that these will be around forever.

- *Financial advisers.* Retirement can be expensive, especially if you
  hope to travel and see the world. Retirement homes cost money
  as well, so if you want to spend your golden years in a place of
  your choice you will need to save the money to do that or you
  may have to settle for something less. A reputable financial
  adviser, either with an investment firm or at your bank, can help
  you set goals and reach them.

- *Investment advice.* Make sure you get good investment advice on
  where to place your RRSPs. Financial advisers, trained bank per-
  sonnel, and insurance agents can all help here, and there are
  endless books you can consult. If you have savings other than
  RRSPs and they are not making any money for you just sitting in
  a savings account, consider investing them in guaranteed investment certificates, savings bonds, mutual funds, or stocks. You
  can invest as little as $100, depending on what you choose.
  Understand your comfort level in choosing investments. If your
  goal is to preserve your assets, while allowing them modest
  growth, you may not want to invest in anything risky. If your goal
  is rapid asset growth, you may be willing to invest some of your
  savings in much riskier ventures for the chance of a big return.
  Ask your bank manager or financial adviser for advice. If your
  assets are large, have your financial adviser point out tax-saving
  devices and investment strategies that will help you and your
  descendants hang on to as much of your hard-earned money as
  possible.

- *Wills.* Make sure you and your spouse both have wills. Otherwise,
  your belongings may not be divided among family members,
  friends, and charities the way you wished. No longer is it permit-
  ted for you to leave everything to one person and cut a son,
  daughter, or wife off completely: the law states that you have cer-

tain obligations. Get a lawyer to help you draw up your will so
that it is legally binding and actually means what you want it to
mean. If you don't wish to pay the $100 or so it costs for a simple
will, do it yourself. Make sure it is in your own handwriting and is
signed and dated. If you type it, you will also need to get the sig-
nature of a witness to ensure its validity in the event of a court
challenge.

- *Living wills.* Consider getting a lawyer to make up a living will for
  you. If you are worried that you may be too ill one day to make
  decisions about your medical care, and if you do not want
  extraordinary measures taken to keep you alive, a living will lets
  both medical staff and family know your wishes. Elsie knew what
  Wayne wanted, but there was no living will, so extraordinary
  measures were taken to keep him alive against his known
  wishes.
- *Lifestyle planning.* Plan ahead emotionally for your retirement.
  Make sure you have something you want to do the day after you
  retire – something that will keep you involved and interested in
  life. Develop new hobbies or plan new adventures *before* you
  retire, and know how you will spend your days.
- *Funeral arrangements.* These can be planned in advance. Alternatively, you can make it known what you want so that the relatives
  you leave behind will know they are doing the right thing at a
  very stressful time. There's nothing worse than family members
  arguing about what their parents wanted, or scrambling around
  trying to find the money to pay for it. The average cost for a
  funeral is $5,000 these days, though much depends on the kind
  of funeral. The estate of a deceased Canadian who had contrib-
  uted to the Canada Pension Plan while alive can recoup up to
  $3,400 of this expense. For details, contact a Canada Pension
  Plan office in your area.
- *General.* As you get older, discuss with your spouse and family
  where you want to live if the home you are in becomes too big,
  or too hard to manage, or if your health begins to deteriorate.
  Also discuss with them your thoughts on in-home care, on being
  cared for by your spouse, on being cared for by your children (in
  your home or their home), and on retirement homes and nurs-

ing homes. Plan ahead, and get yourself on a waiting list and let your family know your plans.

Discuss with your family what should happen if dementia strikes and you can no longer make decisions for yourself. Give power of attorney to your spouse or, failing that, a trusted daughter, son, or friend, so that your affairs can still be handled for you. A lawyer can help you with this.

Review your financial situation every six months or so, and your will every year, and make sure they still reflect what you want.

*   *   *

The tiny balcony of Mum and Dad's new apartment is relatively quiet, and the cool June night air is refreshing after the noise and congestion of the party raging inside. I have escaped for a moment of peace, and from where I sit in the darkness I can see my family milling about inside; each of us is still wearing the flowing black graduation robes that the school lent us for our graduation from our 'planning for the future' course.

I can see David's animated face as he talks to Danielle, probably about his new promotion. He's moving to the East Coast for two years and is on track for upper management. Danielle is just back from her six months abroad – she's the only one not in a black robe, but Peter insisted we enrol her in a summer course before she leaves for Toronto and her first year in kinesiology this fall.

I can hear the phone ringing, and I watch as Bryan comes out of the kitchen to answer it, spatula in hand and a bright floral apron ludicrously pinned around the elegance of his flowing black robe. I can see my parents and Peter sitting on the sofa talking together like three monks. They are probably talking about the Internet. The three of them are hooked and have already settled on what equipment they would like to buy, if they can ever swing the money. Dad is keen to join an Internet discussion group on Beethoven, and Mum wants to follow her modest new investments and correspond by e-mail with her sister in Australia. Peter is, well, still Peter – still a teenager trying to figure out what he wants to do with his life. He's leaning heavily toward financial planning, since he outshone all of us in his exam. Being a teenager, he won't let us forget it. Meanwhile he's interviewing his grandparents and plans to write up their biographies as soon as he can earn the money to buy the computer he says he has to have to do a really professional job.

I look at all the pieces of my family that have placed me smack in the middle of the Sandwich Generation and that make up my particular sandwich and realize with satisfaction that, for us, the good times have far outweighed the bad. Peter and David have developed a relationship with their grandparents that I can only envy, and David has finally found his place in the working world. I have come to understand some of my parents' fears, and our relationship has strengthened and matured into something new and different. At home, Peter still leaves clothes lying around, but he and Bryan are much better at helping out with meals and chores and visiting Mum and Dad. I'll miss David, of course, as I have missed Danielle, but life is a continuum and I realize that all the frightening and exciting potential of the future beckons each one of us in a different way.

'Hey, what are you doing hiding out here?' Bryan's voice startles me out of my reverie, and I turn to greet him. The floral apron is gone, and so is the spatula, and his smile is large enough to light up the darkness of the balcony, and then some.

'Not hiding,' I answer, 'just savouring the moment.'

'Well, the moment's only just begun,' he says, pulling me to my feet, as the strains of Beethoven drift out to us, amid the warm laughter and muffled talk of our family. He releases my hand and bows deeply, swinging his black robe around him like a matador and smiling like Dracula.

'May I have this dance?' he asks.

'But isn't dinner ready?' I ask, laughing.

'God, what a romantic you are, Becca. Dinner can wait, and besides, you need to practise your dancing.'

I cock my eye questioningly at him.

'I just got a very interesting phone call. Remember the raffle ticket I bought?' Before I can answer, he twirls me around in a pirouette.

'We won, Becca. We're going to Montreal for the weekend. Just the two of us!'

Resources

Selected Services for Seniors in Metropolitan Toronto

Call for prices, as they differ from service to service: some are subsidized and some are 'for profit.'

Adult Day Care
Baycrest Centre for Geriatric Care, 789-5131
Villa Colombo Home for the Aged, 789-2113

Practical Assistance
Bernard Betel Centre for Creative Living, 225-2112
Don Mills Foundation for Senior Citizens, 447-7244
Family Service Association of Metropolitan Toronto, 922-3126
Meals on Wheels and More, 492-5811

Audiology Services
Canadian Hearing Society, 964-9595
Sunnybrook Health and Science Centre, 480-6100

Friendly Visiting
Downtown Care-Ring, 868-1190
Victorian Order of Nurses, 499-2009

Letter Carriers Alert
Letter carriers take note of uncollected mail/newspapers and notify contact persons, 979-8822

Snow Removal
City of North York, 395-7300
Toronto, City Hall, 392-7768

Transportation
Toronto Transit Commission – Wheel Trans, 393-4333

Counselling Services for Seniors
Queen Street Mental Health Centre, 535-8501
West Park Hospital, 243-3600
Check with other hospitals.

Miscellaneous
Community Information Centre, 392-0505. Free inquiry service about services in
    Metropolitan Toronto.
Senior Care, 635-2860. Home help, homemaking, friendly visiting, counselling.
Senior Link, 691-7407. Home support services, social and educational programs,
    supportive housing.
Seniors Central Housing Registry, 392-6111. One-stop shopping for seniors look-
    ing for permanent affordable rental housing.
Seniors Repair Service, 752-3866. Seniors on low income – minor home repairs.
Extendicare Canada, 226-1331. Nursing homes for adults 18 years and over.
Second Mile Club of Toronto, 897-0841. Friendly visiting, telephone security
    check.
Wheel Trans, 393-4111. Specialized public transportation.
Sprint, 481-6411. Home visit, Victorian Order of Nurses on premises for assess-
    ment.
Home Care Program for Metropolitan Toronto, 229-2929, 229-5821. Nursing,
    physiotherapy, occupational therapy.

Resources in Your Community

Check your local phone book in the Yellow Pages for services to the elderly under
headings such as these:

1. Senior Citizens Services and Centres. Gives a whole range of services that,
    depending on your community, could include the following:
    Community information centre
    Respite care
    Day care for seniors or eldercare
    Dial-a-ride volunteer drivers
    Family service agencies for counselling
    Foster grandparent programs
    Friendly visitors
    Housing registries for senior housing
    Meals on Wheels

Mobile libraries
Retirement counselling
Senior citizens' centres
Seniors for seniors services
Special clinics for seniors (i.e., foot, hearing, eye)
Volunteers for home repairs
2. Homes – Elderly People
3. Retirement Communities and Homes
4. Home Health Services and Supplies: homemaker's services; nurses, etc.; visiting homemakers, etc.
5. Nurses: visiting nurses, etc.
6. Social Service Organizations: Browse this list! It can be very long and very useful, listing organizations and service clubs ranging from Visiting Homemakers to VON to the Canadian Red Cross, YWCA, Youth Services, Alzheimer's Association, and many more.

If you have access to canada411 (more than 10 million Canadian addresses and phone numbers of businesses, organizations, and individuals) on the Internet, check for countrywide listings at this URL: http://www.canada411.sympatico.ca/. Or simply search for canada411.

National Resources, Profit and Nonprofit

Alzheimer Society of Canada. National office, 1320 Yonge St., Ste. 201, Toronto, ON, M4T 1X2. P: (416) 925-3552, F: (416) 925-1649

The Arthritis Society. National office, 250 Bloor St. E., Ste. 901, Toronto, ON, M4W 3P2. P: (416) 967-1414, F: (416) 967-7171. Nonprofit organization with provincial offices. Dedicated to funding and promoting research on arthritis, public education and patient care

Canadian Cancer Society. Nonprofit organization with branches across the country. National office, 10 Alcorn Ave., Ste. 200, Toronto, ON, M4V 3B1. P: (416) 961-7223, F: (416) 961-4189.

Canadian Home Care Association. National office, 17 York St., Ste 401, Ottawa, ON, K1N 9J6. P: (613) 569-1585, F: (613) 569-1604. National association.

Canadian Red Cross Society. National office, 1800 Alta Vista Dr., Ottawa, ON, K1G 4J5. P: (613) 739-3000, F: (613) 739-2575. Has provincial branches in all provinces. Operates community-based programs such as homemakers', seniors, and veterans' services and equipment loan service.

Canadian Work and Family Services. 155 Gordon Baker Rd., Ste. 201, North York, ON, M2H 3N7. P: 1-800-567-2255, F: (416) 496-8258. Helps employees manage their work and their families by offering services to employers to create supportive work environments.

Childcare Advocacy Association of Canada. National office, 323 Chapel St., Ottawa, ON, K1N 7Z2, P: (613) 594-3196, F: (613) 594-9375. Nonprofit organization promoting high-quality, accessible, affordable child care.

Elderhostel Canada. National office, 308 Wellington St., Kingston, ON, K7K 7A7. P: (613) 530-2222, F: (613) 530-2096, e-mail: ehcadmin@limestone.kosone.com. Nonprofit organization offering low-cost residential education programs for older retired or nearly retired adults in co-operation with more than 350 institutions in Canada.

Extendicare (Canada) Inc. 3000 Steeles Ave. E., Markham, ON, L3R 9W2 P: (905) 470-5545, F: (905) 470-5588. Canada's largest supplier of nursing home care. Also provides management and consulting services and operates retirement homes.

Health Canada. Head office. Ottawa, ON K1A 0K9.

Homesupport Canada, 119 Ross Ave., Ste. 104, Ottawa, ON, K1Y 0N6. P: (613) 761-8609, F: (613) 728-6101. This is an association of agencies and individuals interested in quality home care. HSC provides members with the latest in research, trends, training resources, etc., in home care.

One Voice – The Canadian Seniors Network. 1005–350 Sparks St., Ottawa, ON, K1R 7S8. P: (613) 238-7624, F: (613) 235-4497. Advocacy Group.

Osteoporosis Society of Canada. 33 Laird Dr., Toronto, ON, M4G 2S9. P: (416) 696-BONE, 1-800-463-6842. National nonprofit organization.

Suicide Information and Education Centre. #201, 1615–10th Ave. SW, Calgary, AB, T3C 0J7. Provides information and training on suicide prevention, intervention awareness, and bereavement. P: (403) 245-3900, F: (403) 245-0299.

Victorian Order of Nurses for Canada. 5 Blackburn Ave., Ottawa, ON, K1N 8A2. P: (613) 233-5694, F: (613) 230-4376. National volunteer organization with 75 branches countrywide helping families with health problems. Provides a wide selection of support and community health services.

YWCA of Canada. 80 Gerrard St. E., Toronto, ON, M5B 1G6. P: (416) 593-9886, F: (416) 971-8084. Nonprofit organization with 42 member associations in Canada. Services include advocacy on womens' issues, support groups, health, research, and counselling.

Internet Resources

There is a vast and ever-changing amount of information/advice/statistics at your fingertips on the Internet. The addresses here are only as current as the publication date of this book. Search the Internet for Sandwich Generation/ elders/ seniors/young adults/children/day care/midlife/baby boomers/retirement/ jobs. Also, for specific organizations such as Alzheimer. A few good places to start are listed below:

American Association of Retired Persons
http://www.aarp.org/index.html
Retirement planning, health issues, advocacy groups, research and information, etc.

Baby Boomers Home Page
http://www.netwalk.com/~duchapl/
Nostalgia, trivia, and some relevant information too. Also, chat rooms.

Boomernet
http://www.boomernet.com/boom/index.htm
U.S.-based, information for boomers.

Charity Village homepage
http://www.charityvillage.com/cvhome.html
A guide to charities on the Internet

For a questionnaire on how to choose a nursing home, check
gopher://gopher.gsa.gov:70/11/cic/health

HandiLinks to Baby Boomers
http://www.ahandyguide.com/cat1/b/b613.htm
For those born between 1946 and 1964

Senior citizens, retirement Canada
http://www.clearinghouse.net/
Canadian-based – links to health topics such as diabetes and cancer, and other interesting information.

American National Resources

Aging Network Services – 4400 East-West Highway, Suite 907, Bethesda, MD, 20814, (301) 657-4329. Consultation, linkage, follow-up, long-distance.

Alzheimer's Association – 919 N. Michigan Avenue, Ste. 1000, Chicago, IL, 60611–1676, (312) 335-8700. Resources and local referrals.

American Association of Homes and Services for the Aging – 901 East St. NW, Ste. 500, Washington, DC, 20004–2037, (202) 783-2242. Housing options.

American Health Care Association – 1201 L Street NW, Washington, DC, 20005–4014, (202) 842-4444. Long-term care, nursing homes.

American Self-help Clearinghouse, St Clare's Riverside Medical Centre, 25 Pocono Road, Denville, NJ, 07834, (201) 625-7101. Referrals to local support groups affiliated with particular diseases.

Assisted Living Facility Association of America, 9401 Lee Highway, Ste. 402, Fairfax, VA, 22301, (703) 691-8100. Consumer checklist for evaluating facilities.

Cancer Information Service – 1-800-4-CANCER. Hotline of National Cancer Institute.

Children of Aging Parents – Woodbourne Office Campus, 1609 Woodbourne Road, Ste. 302A, Levittown, PA, 19057, (215) 945-6900. Clearinghouse on caregiver issues, local referrals.

Daughters of Elderly Bridging the Unknown Together (DEBUT), c/o Area 10 Agency on Aging, 2129 Yost Ave., Bloomington, IN, 47403, (812) 876-5319. Support group for women coping with care of aging parents.

Elder Care Locator – 1-800-677-1166, Mon.–Fri. 9:00 a.m.–11:00 p.m., EST. Assistance for seniors.

National Council of Senior Citizens – 1331 F St. NW, Washington, DC, 20004–171, (202) 347-8800. Referrals to long-term care services, nursing homes.

National Family Caregivers Association – 9223 Longbranch Parkway, Silver Springs, MD, 20901–3642, (301) 949-3638. Membership group for caregivers, newsletter.

Statistics

The Sandwich Generation in Canada

- Out of the 9.2 million Canadians aged 35–64, 3.4 million or 37 per cent belonged to the middle layer. In the age group 40–44, the proportion of the middle-layer persons was as high as 58 per cent. Thus, the sandwich family is by no means a marginal phenomenon.
- The mean age of the mid-layer was 43.4 years, with 84 per cent of all cases concentrated in the age bracket 35–49.
- In approximately 1.5 million cases (45 per cent of all mid-layer persons) both parents of the mid-layer were alive; in another 1.5 million cases (44 per cent) only the mother was alive, and in the remaining 360,000 cases (11 per cent) only the father was alive.
- In over half of all cases (55 per cent) the oldest parent was 74 or younger; in only 236,000 cases (7 per cent), did the mid-layer persons have one or two parents aged 85 +.
- A particularly large group of mid-layer persons – 1.7 million, or 52 per cent – had at least one adolescent child (aged 13–18). Adult children (19 +) were found in 1.1 million cases (33 per cent), and of these, 619,000 had adult children only. Relatively few mid-layer persons (5 per cent) had pre-schoolers only (ages 0–4), or pre-schoolers and children in other age groups (10 per cent.) *Source*: Norland, 1994.

America's Senior Sandwich Layer (age 65+)

- 13 per cent of the population is 65 years and older.
- In the year 2030, 22 per cent will be senior citizens.

- there are three million Americans age 85 or older.
- By the year 2030, there will be more Americans over 65 than there are children under 18.
- Today a 65-year-old can expect to live more than 17 additional years.
- In 1994 there were 20 million women and 14 million men over age 65 – a ratio of three to two.
- About 7 million Americans over the age of 65 depend on others for help with activities of daily living.
- A 1992 survey found that almost one in three women and men aged 55 or over serve as informal caregivers. Women spend the most time providing care.
  Source: Brofenbrenner, U., et al. (1996). *The State of Americans*. New York: Free Press.

Notes

Preface / Chapter 1: The Sandwich Generation

1 D. Miller, 'The "Sandwich Generation": Adult Children of the Aging,' *Social Work* 26 (1981) 419–23.
2 J.A. Norland, 'The Sandwich Generation in Canada: Basic Demographic Characteristics,' unpublished paper (Ottawa: Statistics Canada, Demography Division, November 1994).
3 E. Brody, *Women in the Middle: Their Parent Care Years* (New York: Springer, 1990).
4 D. Raphael and B. Schlesinger, 'Women in the Sandwich Generation: Do Adult Children Living at Home Help?' *Journal of Women and Aging* 6 (1/2) (1994): 21–46.
5 J. Dumas and A. Bélanger, *Report on the Demographic Situation in Canada, 1994. The Sandwich Generation: Myths and Reality*, Catalogue #91–209E (Ottawa: Statistics Canada, 1994).
6 'Caregivers of the 1990s,' *Transition* 20 (March), Special Issue. Vanier Institute of the Family.
7 M. Beck 'Aging: Trading Places,' *Newsweek*, 16 July 1990, 48–54.

Chapter 2: Velcro™ Kids

1 B. Okimoto, J. Davies, and P. Stegall, *Boomerang Kids: How to Live with Adult Kids Who Return Home* (Boston: Little Brown, 1987).
2 D. Sunter, 'Youths and the Labour Market,' *Canadian Economic Observer* (Ottawa: Statistics Canada (1997), 3.1–3.7.
3 D. Raphael and B. Schlesinger, 'Women in the Sandwich Generation: Do Adult Children Living at Home Help?' *Journal of Women and Aging* 6(1/2) (1994): 21–46.

4 L. White, 'Co-Residence and Leaving Home: Young Adults and Their Parents,' *Annual Review of Sociology* 20 (1994): 81–102.
5 W.S. Aquilino, 'The Likelihood of Parent–Adult Co-Residence: Effects of Family Structure and Parental Characteristics,' *Journal of Marriage and the Family* 52 (1990): 405–19.
6 W.S. Aquilino and K.R.P. Supple, 'Parent–Child Relations and Parent's Satisfaction with Living Arrangements When Adult Children Live at Home,' *Journal of Marriage and the Family* 53 (1991): 13–27.
7 B. Mitchell and E.M. Gee, 'Boomerang Kids and Mid-Life Parental Satisfaction,' *Family Relations* 45 (1996): 442–8.
8 R. Hartley, 'Paying Board,' *Family Matters* (Australia) 24 (August 1989): 14–16.
9 R. Hartley, 'Young Adults Living at Home,' *Family Matters* (Australia) 36 (December 1993): 35–7.

Chapter 3: The Second Slice of the Sandwich

1 J.A. Mancini and R. Blieszner, 'Aging Parents and Adult Children: Research Themes in Intergenerational Relations,' *Journal of Marriage and the Family* 51 (1989): 275–90.
2 E. Brody, *Women in the Middle: Their Parent Care Years* (New York: Springer, 1990).
3 J.B. Bond, M.R. Baril, S. Axelrod, and L. Crawford, 'Support to Older Parents and Middle Aged Children,' *Canadian Journal of Community Mental Health* 9 (1990): 163–78.
4 I.A. Connidis, *Family Ties and Aging* (Toronto: Butterworths, 1989), 45–70.
5 J. Dumas and A. Bélanger, *Report on the Demographic Situation in Canada 1994. The Sandwich Generation: Myths and Reality,* Catalogue #91–209E (Ottawa: Statistics Canada, 1994).
6 J. Hagey, 'Help Around the House: Support for Older Canadians,' *Canadian Social Trends* (Autumn 1984): 22–4.
7 C. Rosenthal, 'Aging and Intergenerational Relations in Canada,' in V. Marshall (ed.), *Aging in Canada*, 2nd ed. (Toronto: Fitzhenry & Whiteside, 1987), 311–35.
8 G.F. Sanders, J. Walters, and J.E. Montgomery, 'Married Elderly and Their Families,' *Family Perspectives* 18 (1984): 45–52.
9 B. Silverstone and H.K. Hyman, *You and Your Aging Parents* (New York: Pantheon, 1989).
10 B. Schlesinger and D. Raphael, 'The Sandwich Generation. The Jewish Woman in the Middle: Stresses and Satisfactions,' *Journal of Psychology and Judaism* 16(2) (1992): 77–95.
11 D. Raphael and B. Schlesinger, 'Women in the Sandwich Generation: Do

Adult Children Living at Home Help?' *Journal of Women and Aging* 6(1/2) (1994): 21–46.

12 H. Glezer, 'Support and Care Between Generations,' *Family Matters* (Australia), 30 (1991): 44–6.

13 N.L. Chappell and R. Litkenhaus. *Informal Caregivers to Adults in British Columbia*, Joint report of the Centre on Aging, University of Victoria, and the Caregivers Association of British Columbia, 1995.

14 E.M. Brody, 'Parent Care as a Normative Family Stress,' *The Gerontologist* 25(1) (1985): 19–29.

15 V.G. Cicirelli, 'Adult Children and Their Elderly Parents,' in T.H. Brubaker, ed., *Family Relationships in Later Life* (Beverly Hills: Sage, 1983).

16 D. Callahan, *What Do Children Owe Elderly Parents?* The Hastings Center Report, April 1985, 32–7.

17 M. Synott, A. Synott, and L. Connell, 'My Father Became My Son,' unpublished paper, Montreal Ville Marie Social Services, 1990.

18 J. Wright, 'Old Age: Myths and Facts,' *The Senior Volunteer* 44 (Spring 1985).

19 E.S. Johnson and D.L. Spence, 'Adult Children and Their Aging Parents: An Intervention Program,' *Family Relations* 31 (1982): 115–22.

20 J.A. Peterson, 'The Relationships of Middle-aged Children and Their Parents,' in P.K. Ragan, ed., *Aging Parents*. Los Angeles: University of Southern California Press, 1979).

Chapter 4: Life in the Middle

1 J. Dumas and A. Bélanger, *Report on the Demographic Situation in Canada, 1994. The Sandwich Generation: Myths and Reality*, Catalogue #91–209E. Ottawa: Statistics Canada, 1994).

2 G. Spitze and J. Logan, 'More Evidence on Women and Men in the Middle,' *Research on Aging* 12(2) (1990):182–98.

3 L.S. Loomis and A. Booth, 'Multi-generational Caregiving and Well-being: The Myth of the Beleaguered Sandwich Generation,' *Journal of Family Issues* 16(2) (March 1995): 131–48.

4 C.J. Rosenthal, S.H. Matthews, and V.W. Marshall, 'Is Parent Care Normative? The Experience of a Sample of Middle-Aged Women,' *Research on Aging* 11 (1989): 244–60.

5 D.E. Stull, K. Bowman, and V. Smerglia, 'Women in the Middle: A Myth in the Making,' *Family Relations* 43 (1994): 319–24.

6 B. Schlesinger and D. Raphael, 'The Woman in the Middle: The Sandwich Generation Revisited,' *International Journal of Sociology of the Family* 23 (Spring 1993): 77–87.

7 J.A. Norland, 'The Sandwich Generation in Canada: Basic Demographic

Characteristics,' unpublished paper (Ottawa: Statistics Canada, Demography Division, November 1994).

8 L. Kaye and J. Applegate, 'Men as Elder Caregivers: A Response to Changing Families,' *American Journal of Orthopsychiatry* 60 (1990): 86–95.

9 E. Brody, *Women in the Middle: Their Parent Care Years* (New York: Springer, 1990).

10 D. Raphael and B. Schlesinger, 'Women in the Sandwich Generation: Do Adult Children Living at Home Help?' *Journal of Women and Aging* 6(1/2) (1994): 21–46.

11 B. Schlesinger and D. Raphael, 'The Sandwich Generation. The Jewish Woman in the Middle: Stresses and Satisfactions,' *Journal of Psychology and Judaism* 16(2) (1992): 77–95.

12 S. Hunter and M. Sundel, 'Midlife for Women: A New Perspective,' *Affilia* 9(2) (1994): 113–28.

13 N. Underwood et al., 'Mid-Life Panic,' *Maclean's*, 19 August 1991, 30–7.

14 M. Zal, *Caught between Growing Children and Aging Parents* (New York: Plenum, 1992).

15 CARNET, *Work and Family: The Survey* (Guelph, Ont.: Canadian Aging Research Network, University of Guelph, 1993).

16 Ontario's Women's Directorate, *Work and Family* (Toronto: Ministry of Community and Social Services, 1991).

17 B. Silverstone and H.K. Hyman, *You and Your Aging Parents* (New York: Pantheon, 1989).

18 'Failing America's Caregivers: A Status Report on Women Who Care,' *Transition* (March 1990).

19 A. Clemens and L. Axelson, 'The Not So Empty Nest: The Return of the Fledgling Adult,' *Family Relations* 34 (1985): 259–64.

20 B.H. Gotttlieb, E.K. Kelloway, and M. Frabonim, 'Aspects of Elder Care That Place Employees at Risk,' *The Gerontologist* 34 (1994): 815–21.

21 J.A. Mancini and R. Blieszner, 'Aging Parents and Adult Children: Research Themes in Intergenerational Relations,' *Journal of Marriage and the Family* 51 (1989): 275–90.

22 C.L. Barnes, B.A. Given, and C.W. Given, 'Parent Caregivers: A Comparison of Employed and Not Employed Daughters,' *Social Work* 40(3) (1995): 375–83.

23 'Caregivers of the 1990s,' *Transition* 20 (March 1990), Special Issue. Vanier Institute of the Family.

24 S. MacDonald, 'An Aging Canada: Sandwich and Caregiver Dilemmas,' *Perspectives* (Summer 1988).

25 C. Baines, P. Evans, and S. Neysmith, *Women's Caring: Feminist Perspectives on Social Welfare* (Toronto: McClelland & Stewart, 1991).

26 A.J. Walker and C.C. Pratt, 'Daughters' Help to Mothers: Intergenerational Aid versus Caregiving,' *Journal of Marriage and the Family* 53 (1991): 3–12.

27 V.G. Cicirelli, 'Adult Children and Their Elderly Parents,' in T.H. Brubaker, ed., *Family Relationships in Later Life* (Beverly Hills: Sage, 1983).

28 J.M. Crawford et al., 'Factors Affecting Sons' and Daughters' Caregiving to Older Parents.' *Canadian Journal on Aging* 13(4) (1994): 454–69.

29 E.M. Brody, 'Parent Care as a Normative Family Stress,' *The Gerontologist* 25(1) (1985): 19–29.

30 S. McDaniel, 'Emotional Support and Family Contacts of Older Canadians,' in *Canadian Social Trends*, vol. 2 (Toronto: Thompson, 1994), 129–32.

31 D. Miller, 'The "Sandwich Generation": Adult Children of the Aging,' *Social Work* 26 (1981): 419–23.

32 C. Baines, P. Evans, and S. Neysmith, *Women's Caring: Feminist Perspectives on Social Welfare* (Toronto: McClelland & Stewart, 1991).

Chapter 5: Sharing the Caring with Family

1 E. Brody, *Women in the Middle: Their Parent Care Years* (New York: Springer, 1990).

2 K. Dahlin, 'The Sandwich Generation,' *University of Toronto Magazine* 21(1) (Autumn 1993): 6–12.

3 J.M. Crawford et al., 'Factors Affecting Sons' and Daughters' Caregiving to Older Parents,' *Canadian Journal on Aging* 13(4) (1994): 454–69.

4 D. Raphael and B. Schlesinger, 'Caring for Elderly Parents and Children Living at Home: The Sandwich Generation,' *Social Work Research and Abstracts* 29(1) (1993): 3–8.

5 D.E. Gelfand and J.D. McCallum, 'Immigration, the Family, and Female Caregivers in Australia,' *Journal of Gerontological Social Work* 22(3/4) (1994): 41–59.

6 L. Kaye and J. Applegate, 'Men as Elder Caregivers: A Response to Changing Families,' *American Journal of Orthopsychiatry* 60 (1990): 86–95.

7 A.J. Walker, C.C. Pratt, and L. Eddy, 'Informal Caregiving to Aging Family Members,' *Family Relations* 44 (1995): 402–11.

8 A.H. Matthews, 'Balancing Work and Family Responsibilities for the Elderly: Who Cares?' 10th Annual A. Wilson Abernathy Distinguished Lecture. Trinity College, University of Toronto, 1992.

9 A. Matthews, L.D. Campbell, and Gerontology Research Centre, 'Gender Roles, Employment, and Informal care,' unpublished paper, 1994.

10 J.B. Bond, M.R. Baril, S. Axelrod, and L. Crawford, 'Support to Older Parents and Middle Aged Children,' *Canadian Journal of Community Mental Health* 9 (1990): 163–78.

11 P.G. Archbold, 'Impact of Parent Caring on Women,' *Family Relations* 32 (1983): 39–45.

12 B. Schlesinger and D. Raphael, 'The Woman in the Middle: The Sandwich Generation Revisited,' *International Journal of Sociology of the Family* 23 (Spring 1993): 77–87.

13 B. Schlesinger and D. Raphael, 'The Sandwich Generation. The Jewish Woman in the Middle: Stresses and Satisfactions.' *Journal of Psychology and Judaism* 16(2)(1992): 77–95.

14 D. Raphael and B. Schlesinger, 'Women in the Sandwich Generation: Do Adult Children Living at Home Help?' *Journal of Women and Aging* 6(1/2) (1994): 21–46.

15 W.S. Aquilino and K.R.P. Supple, 'Parent–Child Relations and Parent's Satisfaction with Living Arrangements When Adult Children Live at Home,' *Journal of Marriage and the Family* 53 (1991): 13–27.

16 B. Mitchell and E.M. Gee, 'Boomerang Kids and Mid-Life Parental Satisfaction,' *Family Relations* 45 (1996): 442–8.

17 C. Millward, 'Intergenerational Family Support: Help or Hindrance?' *Family Matters* (Australia) 39 (December 1994), 10–13.

18 D. Schlesinger and B. Raphael, 'The Woman in the Middle: The Sandwich Generation Revisited,' *International Journal of Sociology of the Family* 23 (1993): 77–87.

19 W.S. Aquilino, 'The Likelihood of Parent–Adult Co-residence: Effects of Family Structure and Parental Characteristics.' *Journal of Marriage and the Family* 52 (1990): 405–19.

20 B. Schlesinger, 'The "Sandwich Generation": Middle-Aged Families under Stress.' *Canada's Mental Health* 37 (September 1989): 11–14.

21 S. McDaniel, 'Emotional Support and Family Contacts of Older Canadians,' in *Canadian Social Trends*, vol. 2 (Toronto: Thompson, 1994), 129–32.

22 J.F. Robertson, 'Significance of Grandparents: Perceptions of Young Adult Grandchildren,' *The Gerontologist* 16 (1976): 137–46.

Chapter 6: Formal Help Is on the Way

1 T. Chui, 'Canada's Population: Charting into the 21st Century.' *Canadian Social Trends* (Autumn 1996): 3–7.

2 R. Beaujot, E.M. Gee, F. Rajulton, and Z.R. Ravanera, *Family Life over the Life Course* (Ottawa: Statistics Canada, 1995).

3 A.H. Matthews, 'Balancing Work and Family Responsibilities for the Elderly: Who Cares?' 10th Annual A. Wilson Abernathy Distinguished Lecture, Trinity College, University of Toronto, 1992.

4 C. Baines, P. Evans, and S. Neysmith, *Women's Caring: Feminist Perspectives on Social Welfare* (Toronto: McClelland & Stewart, 1991).

5 N.L. Chappell and R. Litkenhaus, *Informal Caregivers to Adults in British Columbia,* Joint report of the Centre on Aging, University of Victoria, and the Caregivers Association of British Columbia, 1995.

Chapter 7: Planning for the Future

1 J.M. Keefe and J.M.M. Blain, *Partnerships in Care: The Involvement of Family Members with Elderly Relatives in Homes for Special Care* (Halifax: Nova Scotia Centre on Aging, Mount Saint Vincent University, 1995).

2 Assisted Living Facility Association of America, 9401 Lee Highway, Suite 402, Fairfax, VA, 22301, (703) 691–8100. Consumer checklist for evaluating facilities. gopher://gopher.gsa.gov:70/00/staff/pa/cic/health/nursehme.xt

3 Office for Senior Citizens Affairs, in co-operation with Ontario Association of Professional Social Workers, *How to Choose the Right Place: A Guide to Services and Facilities for Older People in Ontario* (Toronto: Government of Ontario, Office of Senior Citizens Affairs, 1990).

4 S. MacDonald, 'An Aging Canada: Sandwich and Caregiver Dilemmas.' *Perspectives* (Summer 1988).

5 E. Brody, *Women in the Middle: Their Parent Care Years* (New York: Springer, 1990).

Bibliography

The Young Adults

Amato, P.R., S.J. Rezac, and N. Booth. (1995). 'Helping between Parents and Young Adult Children Offspring: The Role of Parental Marital Quality, Divorce and Remarriage.' *Journal of Marriage and the Family* 57, 363–74. What kind of reciprocal help is there between parents and young adults?

Aquilino, W.S. (1990). 'The Likelihood of Parent–Adult Co-Residence: Effects of Family Structure and Parental Characteristics.' *Journal of Marriage and the Family* 52, 405–19. A sample of 4,893 households was investigated. The authors found that co-residence of young adult children and parents constituted a high percentage of households.

Aquilino, W.S., and K.R.P. Supple. (1991). 'Parent–Child Relations and Parent's Satisfaction with Living Arrangements When Adult Children Live at Home.' *Journal of Marriage and the Family* 53, 13–27. A study of 609 parents whose average age was 51 and young adult children living at home. In most cases the co-residence worked out well.

Boyd, M., and D. Norris. (1989). 'Young Adults Living in Their Parents' Homes.' *Canadian Social Trends* (Summer). A Canadian view of young adults who are remaining longer at home.

– (1995). 'Leaving the Nest? The Impact of Family Structure.' *Canadian Social Trends* (Autumn), 14–16. A statistical analysis of Canada's young adult children who still live at home. About two-thirds of men and women aged 20 to 24 live with a parent.

Boyd, M., and E.T. Pryor. (1990). 'Young Adults Living in Their Parents' Home.' In C. Mckie and K. Thompson, eds., *Canadian Social Trends*. Toronto: Thompson Educational Publishing, 188–95. A statistical profile of the number of young adult children living at home in Canadian families.

– (1994). 'The Cluttered Nest: The Living Arrangements of Young Canadian Adults.' In F. Trovato and C.F. Grindstaff, eds., *Perspectives on Canada's Population*. Toronto: Oxford University Press, 294–306. Canada's young adults will spend more time in a parental setting.

Clemens, A., and L. Axelson. (1985). 'The Not So Empty Nest: The Return of the Fledgling Adult.' *Family Relations* 34, 259–64. A discussion of American trends, in which adult young children return home after an absence of various lengths.

Davis, L. (1996). 'They're Baaack!' *Maturity* (July–August), 12–14. A popular article about boomerang children. The Canadian author includes a guide to successful boomeranging.

Feuerstein, P. (1981). *The Not-So-Empty Nest: How to Live with Your Kids after They've Lived Someplace Else*. Chicago: Folett Publishing. A book full of advice for parents with boomerang children.

Grindstaff, C.E. (1996). 'Canadian Fertility: From Boom to Bust or Stability.' *Canadian Social Trends* (Winter), 12–16. A demographic analysis of various Canadian age cohorts.

Hartley, R. (1989). 'Paying Board.' *Family Matters* (Australia) 24 (August), 14–16. A study on employed young adult children who remain home longer. Are they paying board? How much are they paying? What are the expectations of parents and children?

– (1993). 'Young Adults Living at Home.' *Family Matters* (Australia) 36 (December), 35–7. An Australian view of young adults living at home.

Kilmartin, C. (1987). 'Leaving Home Is Coming Later.' *Family Matters* 9 (October), 40–2. When do young adult children leave home, and why are they staying at home longer?

Mitchell, B., and E.M. Gee. (1996). 'Boomerang Kids and Mid-Life Parental Satisfaction.' *Family Relations* 45, 442–8. A study of 172 parents of boomerang kids in British Columbia. The overall marital satisfaction of the parents is quite high (73% were satisfied).

Mitchell, B.A., A.V. Wister, and T.K. Burch. (1989). 'The Family Environment and Leaving the Parental Home.' *Journal of Marriage and the Family* 51, 605–13. This Canadian sample included 14,004 respondents between the ages of 18 and 64. It examines when children leave home in various types of families.

Okimoto, B., J. Davies, and P. Stegall. (1987). *Boomerang Kids: How to Live with Adult Kids Who Return Home*. Boston: Little Brown. A book of advice for parents who find that their young adult children have returned home.

Quinn, J.B. (1993). 'What's for Dinner, Mom?' *Newsweek*, 5 April, p. 68. A pungent column about America's boomerang generation, consisting of 11 million young adult children who return home.

Steckel, R.H. (1996). 'The Age at Leaving Home in the United States, 1850–

1860.' *Social Science History* 20(4) (Winter), 507–32. A historical study which indicates that young adults left home in their early to mid-twenties.

Sunter, D. 1997. 'Youths and the Labour Market.' *Canadian Economic Observer* (May). Ottawa: Statistics Canada. 3.1–3.7. The reasons why many young adult children are staying home are related to the economic situation in Canada.

Tourfexis, A. (1987). 'Show Me the Way to Go Home.' *Time* 4 May. Case histories of young adult children who are living with their parents.

Usher, C.M. (1995). *Boomerang Kids: When Adult Children Return Home.* Vancouver: B.C. Council for the Family. This pamphlet has a good description of boomerang children, including a contract you can make with the young adult child. (204–2590 Granville Street, Vancouver, BC, V6H 3H1.)

Veevers, J.E., and B.A. Mitchell. (1994). 'Intergenerational Perceptions of Support: A Comparison of "Boomerang" Kids and Their Parents.' Unpublished paper, presented at the Annual Meeting of the Canadian Sociology and Anthropology Association, Calgary, June 10–14. A sample of 218 Canadian families with children who returned home. What effects do the boomerang children have on their parents?

White, L. (1994). 'Co-Residence and Leaving Home: Young Adults and Their Parents.' *Annual Review of Sociology* 20, 81–102. An American study which illustrates that co-residence of young adult children and parents can have positive results.

Wiener, V. (1997). *The Nesting Syndrome.* Minneapolis: Fairview. This book discusses the increasing phenomenon of adult children living at home and returning to their homes (the nesters). It is a popular book of advice that focuses on the United States.

The Middle Layer

American Association of Retired Persons. (1995). Caregiver Resource Kit. Washington, D.C.: AARP. A useful kit that contains important information for caregivers, including useful resources for Americans. (Free of charge: 6011 East Street, N.W., Washington, DC, 20049.)

Aranda, M.P., and B.G. Knight. (1997). 'The Influence of Ethnicity and Culture on the Caregiver Stress and Coping Process: A Sociocultural Review and Analysis.' *The Gerontologist* 37(3), 342–54. A review of the literature on ethnic minority caregivers that focuses on Latinos.

Archbold, P.G. (1983). 'Impact of Parent Caring on Women.' *Family Relations* 32, 39–45. A discussion of the stressors confronted by women who have some caring responsibilities for their parents.

Aronson, J. (1991). 'Dutiful Daughters and Undemanding Mothers: Constraining Images of Giving and Receiving Care in Middle and Later Life.' In C.T. Baines,

P.M. Evans, and S.M. Neysmith, eds., *Women's Caring: Feminist Perspectives on Social Welfare.* Toronto: McClelland & Stewart, 138–68. In Canada, 85 to 90 per cent of the care of elderly persons is provided informally by their families. Mostly women are the care providers. Case studies illustrate the work of the 'caretaker.'

Barnes, C.L., B.A. Given, and C.W. Given. (1994). 'Parent Caregivers: A Comparison of Employed and Not Employed Daughters.' *Social Work* 40(3), 375–83. An examination of the stresses of employed and not employed daughters.

Bass, D.S. (1990). *Caring Families, Supports and Interventions.* Silver Spring, MD: NASW Press. This book deals with issues of caregiving, and suggests ways of dealing with them so that caregiving is a little easier. (National Association of Social Workers, 7981 Eastern Avenue, Silver Spring, MD, 20910.)

Beck, M. (1992). 'The New Middle Age.' *Newsweek,* 7 December, 50–7. A discussion of middle age in the 1990s.

Bennett, J.M., M. Dellmann-Jenkins, and D. Lambert. (1996). 'Adult Sons as the Primary Family Member Providing Support to Older Institutionalized Parents.' *Family Perspective* 30(1), 5–20. One of the few items that focuses on males who provide elder care.

Brody, E. (1990). *Women in the Middle: Their Parent Care Years.* New York: Springer. A classic book that describes in detail some of the issues facing the 'woman in the middle' of the sandwich.

Callahan, D. (1985). 'What Do Children Owe Elderly Parents?' The Hastings Center Report, April, 32–7. An essay that questions the responsibilities that adult children have toward their parents in North America.

'Caregivers of the 1990s.' (1990). *Transitions* 20 (March). Special Issue. Vanier Institute of the Family. A special issue devoted to caregivers of the 1990s.

CARNET. (1993). *Work and Family: The Survey.* The Canadian Aging Research Network. A Canadian study of 5,121 respondents from eight organizations. The findings were related to elder care of employees in these organizations. Forty-six per cent were involved in elder care.

Crawford, J.M., et al. (1994). 'Factors Affecting Sons' and Daughters' Caregiving to Older Parents.' *Canadian Journal on Aging* 13(4), 454–69. What are some of the effects of caring for elder parents on sons and daughters?

Dahlin, K. (1993). 'The Sandwich Generation.' *University of Toronto Magazine* 21(1) (Autumn), 6–12. A popular article on the Sandwich Generation.

DeVaus, D. (1996). 'Children's Responsibilities to Their Elderly Parents.' *Family Matters* (Australia) 45 (Summer), 16–21. A national Australian sample of 2,129 randomly selected adults were surveyed about responsibility for older parents.

Dumas, J. and A. Bélanger. (1994). *Report on the Demographic Situation in Canada 1994. The Sandwich Generation: Myths and Reality.* Ottawa: Statistics Canada, Catalogue #91–209E. A detailed analysis of the demographic Canadian trends related to the Sandwich Generation. (Marketing Sales and Service, Statistics Canada, Ottawa, Ontario, K1A OT6).

Eckert, J.W., and S.C. Shulman. (1996). 'Daughters Caring for Their Aging Mothers: A Midlife Developmental Process.' *Journal of Gerontological Social Work* 25(3/4), 17–32. This paper examines the developmental crisis for women in midlife when caring for an aging parent, based on clinical experiences in outpatient settings.

'Failing America's Caregivers.' (1990). *Transitions* (March). A status report on women who care. How do family caregivers manage?

Farkas, J.I., and C.L. Hymes. (1997). 'The Influence of Caregiving and Employment on the Voluntary Activities of Midlife and Older Women.' *Journal of Gerontology: Social Sciences* 52B, 4,S-180-S-189. Caregivers use outside voluntary activities as a way to relieve the stress caused by caregiving tasks. They are able to balance various roles.

Gallagher, W. (1993). 'Myths of Middle Age.' *The Atlantic* 27(1) (May), 51–83. Middle age may be the best time of your life, researchers discover. An excellent article on this part of the life cycle.

Gignac, M.A.M., E.K. Kelloway, and B.H. Gottlieb. (1996). 'The Impact of Caregiving on Employment: A Mediational Model of Work-Family Project.' *Canadian Journal on Aging* 15, 525–42. A survey of 714 employees in eight organizations examined their elder care responsibilities. Conflict between family and work was also investigated.

Gelfand, D.E., and J.D. McCallum. (1994). 'Immigration, the Family, and Female Caregivers in Australia.' *Journal of Gerontological Social Work* 22(3/4), 41–59. The impact of Australian immigration on first-generation immigrant women who are providing care for their parents.

Guberman, N. (1990). 'The Family, Women and Caregiving: Who Cares for the Caregivers?' In V. Dhruvarja ed., *Women and Well-Being*. Montreal: McGill-Queen's University Press, 67–77. We forget that caregivers need a lot of support. This paper raises the issues related to who 'cares for the caregivers.'

Hagen, B., and E. Gallagher. (1996). 'Looking Out for Family Caregivers.' *The Canadian Nurse* 92(3), 27–31. Offering family caregivers education and support can be nothing short of 'life saving' for them. A discussion of the use of caregivers' groups in British Columbia.

Hartley, R. (1990). 'The Never-Empty Nest.' *Family Matters* (Australia) 26, 67–9. An Australian study of the Sandwich Generation.

Himes, C.L. (1994). 'Parental Caregiving by Adult Women: A Demographic Perspective,' *Research on Aging* 16(2), 191–211. An American demographic analysis of 3,543 adult white women who have eldercare responsibilities. Daughters

are traditional sources of assistance in the care of elderly parents. This study
examines the practice of parental care over the life of adult women.

Hunter, S. and M. Sundel. (1994). 'Midlife for Women: A New Perspective.' *Affilia*
9(2), 113–28. A feminist analysis of the midlife of women today.

Kaye, L., and J. Applegate. (1990). 'Men as Elder Caregivers: A Response to
Changing Families.' *American Journal of Orthopsychiatry* 60, 86–95. One of the
few papers that discusses men as caregivers.

Klingelhofer, E.L. (1989). *Coping with Grown Children.* New York: Dell. How to
relate to grown-up children.

Loomis, L.S., and A. Booth. (1995). 'Multi-generational Caregiving and Well-
Being: The Myth of the Beleaguered Sandwich Generation. *Journal of Family
Issues* 16(2) (March), 131–48. An American sample of 2,033 married persons
between the ages of 16 and 55 years were interviewed by telephone. Some of
the findings include the fact that 'strong marriages' help alleviate the stressors
of the Sandwich Generation.

MacDonald, S.A. (1988). An Aging Canada: Sandwich and Caregiver Dilemmas.
Perspectives, 12(1), 15–18. Addressed to nurses, the paper examines caregiving
dilemmas. Canadian demographic trends are also included.

MacLean, H. (1987). *Caring for Your Parents.* New York: Doubleday. A book of
advice for those who care for their parents.

Matthews, A.H. (1992). 'Balancing Work and Family Responsibilities for the
Elderly: Who Cares?' 10th Annual A. Wilson Abernathy Distinguished Lecture,
Trinity College, University of Toronto. What initiatives have some companies
taken to help employees with elder care?

Matthews, A., L.D. Campbell, and Gerontology Research Centre. (1994.)
'Gender Roles, Employment and Informal Care.' Unpublished paper, University of Guelph. A look at the dual roles of employment and caregiving for
women.

Miller, D. (1981). 'The "Sandwich Generation": Adult Children of the Aging.'
Social Work 26, 419–23. The pioneering paper that sets out the family issues associated with the Sandwich Generation.

McDaniel, S. (1994). 'Emotional Support and Family Contacts of Older
Canadians.' In *Canadian Social Trends.* Vol. 2. Toronto: Thompson, 129–32.
Spouses and adult children are the main sources of emotional support for most
Canadians aged 65 and over in 1990. (14 Ripley Avenue, Ste. 105, Toronto,
Ontario, M6S 3N9.)

McKibbon, J., L. Genereux, and G. Seguin-Roberge. (1996). 'Who Cares for the
Caregivers?' *The Canadian Nurse* 92(3), 38–41. An important article which
reminds us that caregivers need support, due to the many stresses they
experience.

Norland, J.A. (1994). 'The Sandwich Generation in Canada: Basic Demographic Characteristics.' Ottawa: Statistics Canada, Demography Division, November, unpublished paper. This paper documents Canadian family statistics related to the Sandwich Generation.

Norris, J. (ed.). (1988). *Daughters of the Elderly: Building Partnerships in Caregiving.* Bloomington: Indiana University Press. Addressed to daughters who have caregiving responsibilities.

Pavalko, E.K., and J.E. Artis. (1997). 'Women's Caregiving and Paid Work: Casual Relationships in Late Midlife.' *Journal of Gerontology: Social Sciences* 528(4), S170–9. Middle-aged women who work and are caregivers are likely to reduce employment hours or stop work because of their caregiving duties.

Raphael, D., and B. Schlesinger. (1993). 'Caring for Elderly Parents and Children Living at Home: The Sandwich Generation.' *Social Work Research and Abstracts* 29(1), 3–8. A report on the statistical methodology of a study of 60 'women in the middle' in Metropolitan Toronto.

Raphael, D., and B. Schlesinger. (1994). 'Women in the Sandwich Generation: Do Adult Children Living at Home Help?' *Journal of Women and Aging* 6(12), 21–46. A summary of the first Canadian study of 66 'women in the middle' of the Sandwich Generation.

Richardson, L., V. Bengtson, and S.R. Miller. (1989). '"The Generation in the Middle." Perceptions of Change in Adults' Intergenerational Relationships.' In K. Krepper and R.M. Lerner, eds., *Family System and Life Span Developments.* Hillsdale, NJ: Erlbaum, 341–66. A research study of middle-aged adults.

Robison, J., P. Moen, and D. Dempster-McClain. (1995). 'Women's Caregiving: Changing Profiles and Pathways.' *Journal of Gerontology,* Series B (50B) (November), S362–73. How do women become caregivers to their aged parents?

Rosenthal, C.J. (1987). 'Family Supports in Later Life: Does Ethnicity Make a Difference?' *The Gerontologist* 26, 19–24. We have a lack of studies on ethnicity and family supports in later life. Various ethnic groups may have different approaches to elder care.

Rosenthal, C.J., S.H. Matthews, and V.W. Marshall. (1989). 'Is Parent Care Normative? The Experience of a Sample of Middle-Aged Women.' *Research on Aging* 11, 244–60. The authors point out that not all middle-aged women are caring for their parents.

Rosenthal, C.J., M. Matthews, and S.H. Matthews. (1996). 'Caught in the Middle? Occupancy in Multiple Roles and Help to Parents in a National Probability Sample of Canadian Adults.' *Journal of Gerontology, Social Sciences* 51B, S274-83. A sample of 2,703 women and 2,412 men in the age range 35–64 and living in Canada were surveyed by telephone. They were asked how typical the experience was of being 'caught in the middle.'

Schlesinger, B. (1989). 'The "Sandwich Generation": Middle-Aged Families
under Stress.' *Canada's Mental Health* 37 (September), 11–14. A summary of
the various layers in the Sandwich Generation. Implications for research are
included.

Schlesinger, B., and D. Raphael. (1992). 'The Sandwich Generation. The Jewish
Woman in the Middle: Stresses and Satisfactions.' *Journal of Psychology and
Judaism* 16(2), 77–95. Among a study of 66 'women in the middle,' there were
ten Jewish women. The paper focuses on the responses of this group.

– (1993). 'The Woman in the Middle: The Sandwich Generation Revisited.'
International Journal of Sociology of the Family 23 (Spring), 77–87. A comprehen-
sive report of the findings of a Canadian study of 66 women who are in the
Sandwich Generation.

Shapiro, B.A., V. Konover, and A. Shapiro. (1993). *The Big Squeeze: Balancing the
Needs of Aging Parents, Dependent Children and You.* New York: Ballantine. A popular book about caregivers who are looking after children at home as well as
aging parents.

Smith, G.C., M.F. Smith, and R.W. Toseland. (1991). 'Problems Identified by
Family Caregivers in Counselling.' *The Gerontologist* 31, 15–21. A study of 51
caregiving women who went for counselling. Case examples illustrate this
paper.

Smith, K. (1989). 'Serving the Sandwich Generation: Working with Adult
Children of Aging Parents.' *Journal of Independent Social Work* 3(3) (Spring), 79–
94. Members of the Sandwich Generation are increasingly seeking professional
help. The paper describes an eight-week workshop–support group for adult
children of aging parents.

Spitze, G. and J. Logan. (1990). 'More Evidence on Women and Men in the Middle.' *Research on Aging* 12(2), 182–98. A description of what happens to men
and women in the middle.

Statistics Canada. (1997). 'Who Cares? Caregiving in the 1990s.' *The Daily*.
29 August, 4–5. A report on women and men who are caregivers in Canada. Of
all the women who lived with a spouse and children, 16 per cent were caregivers to elderly parents. The largest percentage of caregivers were women in the
45–64 age group.

Stull, D.E., K. Bowman, and V. Smerglia. (1994). 'Women in the Middle: A Myth
in the Making.' *Family Relations* 43, 319–24. A study of 'women in the middle.'
Employment outside the home was related to an increase in physical strain in
caregiving. The presence of children in the home did not create too much
stress.

Suitor, J.J., and K. Pillemer. (1987). 'The Presence of Adult Children: A Source of
Stress for Elderly Couples' Marriages.' *Journal of Marriage and the Family* 49,

717–25. This study points out that the presence of adult children provides stressors for elderly couples. Other studies disagree with these findings.

Tebb, S. (1995). 'An Aid to Empowerment: A Caregiver Well-Being Scale.' *Health and Social Work* 20, 87–92. A simple valid scale was developed to assess the extent to which a caregiver's basic human needs are being met.

Tully, S. (1997) 'Caring for the Caregiver.' *Perspectives: Journal of the Gerontological Nursing Association* 21(2) (Summer), 5–8. Caring for elderly parents can cause stress at home and at work. Employees should take eldercare into consideration.

Underwood, N., et al. (1991). 'Mid-Life Panic.' *Maclean's*, 19 August 1991, 30–7. A popular look at Canadians in midlife.

Walker, A.J., and K.R. Allen. (1991). 'Relationships between Caregiving Daughters and their Elderly Mothers.' *The Gerontologist* 31(3), 389–96. A study of 29 pairs of widowed mothers and their caregiving daughters. Social exchange theory is tested out in this relationship.

Walker, A.J., and C.C. Pratt. (1991). 'Daughters' Help to Mothers: Intergenerational Aid Versus Caregiving.' *Journal of Marriage and the Family* 53, 3–12. Significant aid is given by daughters to their mothers. This includes instrumental and psychological aid.

Walker, A.J., C.C. Pratt, and L. Eddy. (1995). 'Informal Caregiving to Aging Family Members.' *Family Relations* 44, 402–11. What is family caregiving? What are its outcomes? What is its relationship to formal caregiving? A review of the literature related to these three questions.

Walker, A.J., C.C. Pratt, and N.C. Oppy. (1992). 'Perceived Reciprocity in Family Caregiving.' *Family Relations* 41, 82–5. A study of 174 care receiving mothers and their caregiving daughters. The majority perceived that daughters received aid from mothers in return for help given.

Wise, G.W., and V.M. Murray. (1987). 'The Empty Nest: The Silent Invasion on Two Fronts.' *Journal of Home Economics* (Spring), 49–53. In the middle years two stages of the family life cycle occur; one is the 'launching centre' and the other is the 'empty nest.' Today the middle years are the 'caught generation,' or the 'Sandwich Generation.'

Zal, M. (1992). *Caught between Growing Children and Aging Parents.* New York: Plenum Press. A psychiatrist discusses the stresses of the Sandwich Generation.

The Elders

Beck. M., et al. (1990). 'Aging. Trading Places.' *Newsweek*, 16 July 1990, 48–54. A lengthy examination of women on the 'daughter track': working, raising children, and helping elderly parents.

Bond, J.B., M.R. Baril, S. Axelrod, and L. Crawford. (1990). 'Support to Older

Parents and Middle Aged Children.' *Canadian Journal of Community Mental Health* 9, 163–78. Evidence shows that adult children act as responsible care-givers in Canadian society. Adult daughters tend to be the major helpers.

Chalam-Zukewich, N. (1996). 'Living with Relatives.' *Canadian Social Trends* (Autumn), 20–4. In 1991 in Canada, 3 per cent of the total population lived with relatives. This is most common among seniors. Six per cent of seniors aged 65–74 lived with relatives.

Chappell, N.L., and R. Litkenhaus. (1995). *Informal Caregivers to Adults in British Columbia.* Joint report of the Centre on Aging, University of Victoria, and the Caregivers Association of British Columbia. A study of informal caregivers in British Columbia.

Cicirelli, V.G. (1983). 'Adult Children and Their Elderly Parents.' In T.H. Brubaker, ed., *Family Relationships in Later Life.* Beverly Hills: Sage. A review of the literature on the relationships between adult children and their elderly parents.

Connidis, I.A. (1989). *Family Ties and Aging.* Toronto: Butterworths, 45–70. A Canadian author writes about the importance of family relationships with the elderly.

Edinberg, M.A. (1987). *Talking with Your Aging Parents.* Boston: Shamshala. How to communicate with elderly parents.

'Family Support of the Elderly: Cross-National Perspectives.' (1983). *The Gerontologist* 23 (December), Special Issue. This special issue reviews family support of the elderly in seven countries.

Glicksman, A. (1990). 'The New Jewish Elderly.' *Journal of Aging and Judaism* 5(1), 7–22. A review of the literature related to Jewish elderly.

Hagey, J. (1989). 'Help Around the House: Support for Older Canadians.' *Canadian Social Trends* (Autumn) 22–4. What kind of help is given to Canada's elderly in their own homes?

Johnson, E.S., and D.L. Spence. (1982). 'Adult Children and Their Aging Parents: An Intervention Program.' *Family Relations* 31, 115–22. A description of an intervention program that attempts to enhance relationships between elderly parents and their adult children.

Jones, M. (1990). 'Time Use of the Elderly.' *Canadian Social Trends* (Summer), 28–30. How do Canada's seniors spend their time, including family care?

Keefe, J.M., and Blain, J.M.M. (1995). Partnerships in Care: The Involvement of Family Members with Elderly Relatives in Homes for Special Care. Halifax: Nova Scotia Centre on Aging, Mount Saint Vincent University.A study of 214 Nova Scotia families who had an elderly family member in an institution. (Mount Saint Vincent University, Halifax, Nova Scotia, B3M 2J6).

Klingelhofer, E.L. (1989). *Coping With Your Grown Children.* New York: Dell. This book gives advice on how to handle 'adult children.'

Lester, A.D., and Lester, J.L. (1980). *Understanding Aging Parents.* Philadelphia: Westminster Press. A helpful book for those who have elderly parents and parents-in-laws.

Mall, J. (1990). *Caregiving: How to Care for your Elderly Mother and Stay Sane.* New York: Ballantine. How to manage stressors as an eldercare person.

Mancini, J.A., and R. Blieszner. (1989). 'Aging Parents and Adult Children: Research Themes in Intergenerational Relations.' *Journal of Marriage and the Family* 51, 275–90. A comprehensive literature review dealing with intergenerational relationships.

Nemeth. M. (1994). 'Amazing Greys: The Sandwich Generation.' *Maclean's,* 10 January, 26–36. An examination of the various layers in the Sandwich Generation, including the elderly layer.

Office for Senior Citizens Affairs in co-operation with Ontario Association of Professional Social Workers. (1990). *How to Choose the Right Place: A Guide to Services and Facilities for Older People in Ontario.* Looking for a place for your elderly parents? A list of available facilities up to 1990.

Ragan, P.K., ed. (1979). *Aging Parents.* Los Angeles: University of Southern California Press. A good collection of articles on the lives of elderly parents.

Robertson, J.F. (1976). 'Significance of Grandparents: Perceptions of Young Adult Grandchildren.' *The Gerontologist* 16, 137–46. How do young adult grandchildren view their grandparents? An important pioneering study.

Sanders, G.F., J. Walters, and J.E. Montgomery. (1984). 'Married Elderly and their Families.' *Family Perspectives* 18, 45–52. A study of 68 elderly married couples whose mean age was 70 years. All couples lived on their own. The study examined their family relationships.

Silverstone, B., and H.K. Hyman. (1989). *You and Your Aging Parents.* New York: Pantheon. A practical guide on dealing with elderly parents.

Synott, M., A. Synott, and L. Connell. 1990. 'My Father Became My Son.' Unpublished paper. Montreal Ville Marie Social Services. Role reversals sometimes occur when adult children have to look after elderly parents.

Watt, J. (1994). *A Caregiver's Guide: Practical Solutions for Coping with Aging Parents or a Chronically Ill Partner or Relative.* 2nd ed. North Vancouver: International Self Counsel. A self-help guide for those who are caregivers to their elderly relatives.

Wright, J. 'Old Age: Myths and Facts.' (1985). *The Senior Volunteer* 44 (Spring). Myths and facts about old age

General Interest

Baines, C., P. Evans, and S. Neysmith. (1991). *Women's Caring: Feminist Perspectives on Social Welfare.* Toronto: McClelland & Stewart. This collection of papers examines the connection between caring and poverty, wife abuse, and child neglect. What are the prevailing assumptions made about caring?

Baker, H., ed. (1996). *Families' Changing Trends in Canada.* Toronto: McGraw-Hill Ryerson. Canadian family life.

Beaujot, R., E.M. Gee, F. Rajulton, and Z.R. Ravanera. (1995). *Family Life over the Life Course.* Ottawa: Statistics Canada. Selected family trends in Canadian society are discussed in this monograph, including family patterns in midlife.

Billig, N. (1995). *Growing Older and Wiser.* New York: Lexington. A geriatric psychiatrist explains how seniors can cope with the normal aging process. A good book for elderly parents.

Blieszner, R., and J.M. Alley. (1996). 'Family Caregiving of the Elderly: An Overview of Resources.' *Family Relations* 39, 97–102. A review of the impact of caregiving on families. Includes a resource section on books, articles, organizations, and programs.

Blieszner, R., and V. Hilkevich. eds. (1995). *Handbook of Aging and the Family.* Westport, CT: Greenwood. Relevant research findings related to aging in the context of family life. This is a multidisciplinary group of papers. A comprehensive overview of the field.

Brody, E.M. (1985). 'Parent Care as a Normative Family Stress.' *The Gerontologist* 25(1), 19–29. A discussion of parent care for women of middle age and the stresses they face.

Bronfenbrenner, V., P. McClelland, E. Wethington, P. Moen, and S.I. Ceci. (1996). *The State of Americans.* New York: Free Press. An easy-to-read guide to the most reliable facts and statistics on diverse topics related to American society.

Brubaker, T.H., eds. (1983). *Family Relationships in Later Life.* Beverly Hills, CA: Sage. Fourteen papers discuss various aspects of family relationships in later life.

Chui, T. (1996). 'Canada's Population: Charting into the 21st Century.' *Canadian Social Trends* (Autumn), 3–5. A demographic profile of Canada's population in the millennium. Population projections include the growth of seniors and the effects on the total population, including the Sandwich Generation.

DeVaus, D. (1994). *Letting Go: Relationships between Adults and Their Parents.* Melbourne: Oxford University Press. An Australian study of the relationships between adults and their parents. Includes numerous case examples.

Driedger, L., and N. Chappell. (1987). *Aging and Ethnicity: Toward an Interface.* Toronto: Butterworths. This monograph looks at Canada's aging population with ethnic roots. Many ethnic families find themselves in the Sandwich Generation.

Eldercare: A Newsletter for Family Members Caring for Elderly Relatives. (Eldercare, 12 Donora Drive, Suite 202, Toronto, Ontario, M4B 1B4; Fax (416) 751–5876.)

Elkind, D. (1994). *Ties that Stress: The New Family Imbalance.* Cambridge: Harvard

University Press. A critical examination of American family life today. Some of the topics include family ties and family values.

Foot, D.K., and D. Stoffman. (1996). *Boom, Bust, and Echo*. Toronto: Macfarlane Walter & Ross. A demographic view of population changes in Canada, including the Sandwich Generation. If we understand changing demographics, we can understand changing family patterns.

Gardner, B. (1996). 'Caregiving: A Man's Job?' *Maturity* (September/October), 25–6. A popular article that examines male caregivers, with case examples.

Gonyea, J.G., ed. (1994). 'Work and Elder Care.' *Research on Aging* 16(1) (March). Special Issue. Five papers discuss work/family conflict related to elder care. The intersection of work and elder care roles is examined.

Joseph, A.E., and B.C. Hallman. (1996). 'Caught in the Triangle: The Influence of Home, Work, and Elder Location on Work–Family Balance.' *Canadian Journal of Aging* 15, 393–412. An examination of 595 employed caregivers who provide assistance to their elderly relatives.

Kosberg, J.I., ed. (1992). *Family Care of the Elderly: Social and Cultural Changes.* Newbury Park, CA: Sage. Seventeen papers discuss family care of the elderly in sixteen countries.

Lustbader, W., and N.R. Hooyman. (1994). *Taking Care of Aging Family Members.* New York: Free Press. A guide for family members on the complete range of psychological, social, and financial issues that face caregivers of older persons.

Marks, N.F. (1996). 'Caregiving Across the Lifespan: National Prevalence and Predictions.' *Family Relations* 45, 27–36. An American survey of 13,107 households. One in 5 women aged 35–64 reported caring for relatives.

Marshall, V., ed. (1987). *Aging in Canada: Social Perspectives.* Toronto: Fitzhenry & Whiteside. A good collection of papers dealing with diverse aspects of aging in Canada.

McMaster University. (1996). *Focus on Aging in Canada.* Hamilton: Office of Gerontological Studies. A comprehensive demographic profile of the elderly (65+) population in Canada. A unique reference tool for studying this age cohort.

Michaels, E. (1995). *Look to This Day: A Complete Guide to Health and Well-Being in Your Later Years.* Toronto: Key Porter. A down-to-earth guide to healthier aging. It makes a good present for parents.

Millward, C. (1994). 'Intergenerational Family Support: Help or Hindrance?' *Family Matters* (Australia), 39 (December), 10–13. Can we assume that close involvement with family necessarily assists in mutual support and exchange?

Moen, P., J. Robinson, and D. Dempster-McClain. (1995). 'Caregiving and Women's Well-being: A Life Course Approach.' *Journal of Health and Social Behavior* 36 (September), 259–73. A random sample of 293 women were interviewed in 1956 and 1986. What women bring to caregiving shapes its significance for their emotional health.

Moore, E.G., M.W. Rosenberg, and D. McGuinness. (1997). *Growing Old in Canada: Demographic and Geographic Perspectives.* Toronto: Nelson. This book explores older Canadians' lives today and tomorrow. It is a monograph produced by Statistics Canada as part of the 1991 Census Program.

National Film Board of Canada. (1994). *The Caring Collection Catalogue.* More than 100 videos related to aspects of caring.

Neugarten, B.L. (1979). The Middle Generations. In P.K. Regan, ed., *Aging Parents.* Los Angeles: University of Southern California Press, 258–66. A description of the personal characteristics related to elderly parents.

Norris, J.E., and J.A. Tindale. (1994). *Among Generations: The Cycle of Adult Relationships.* New York: W.H. Freeman. This book discusses the complex cycle of family relationships from generation to generation.

Ontario's Women's Directorate. (1991). *Work and Family.* Toronto: Ministry of Community and Social Services. A booklet about the tensions of work and family encountered by women.

Owram, D. (1996). *Born at the Right Time: A History of the Baby Boom Generation.* Toronto: University of Toronto Press. Canada's baby boomers will also move into the Sandwich Generation. A fascinating historical look at this cohort from the end of the Second World World War to the close of the 1960s.

Paro-Med Health Services. (1996). *Canadian Attitudes about Home Health Services.* Toronto: Paro-Med Health Services. Report.

Peorlin, L.I., J.T. Mullan, S.J. Semple, and M.M. Skaff. (1990). 'Caregiving and the Stress Process: An Overview of Concepts and Their Measures.' *The Gerontologist* 30(5), 583–91. An examination of the stresses that affect caregivers, and how one can measure these stressors.

Peterson, J.A. (1979). 'The Relationships of Middle-Aged Children and Their Parents.' In P.K. Ragan, ed. *Aging Parents.* Los Angeles: University of Southern California Press. Review article on relationships between parents and their middle-aged children.

Robinson, J., P. Moen, and D. Dempster-McClain. (1995). 'Women's Caregiving: Changing Profiles and Pathways.' *Journal of Gerontology: Social Sciences* S362–73. Women with more traditional lifestyles are more like to become caregivers. This article looks at various pathways to caregiving.

Rosenthal, C. (1987). 'Aging and Intergenerational Relations in Canada.' In V. Marshall, ed. *Aging in Canada.* 2nd ed. Toronto: Fitzhenry & Whiteside, 311–35. Research has destroyed the myth that elder persons are isolated from and abandoned by their families.

Schlesinger, R., and B. Schlesinger. (1992). *Canadian Families in Transition.*

Toronto: Canadian Scholars' Press. This book includes changes in various patterns of Canadian families in the 1990s. The Sandwich Generation is included.

Cross-Cultural References

Braun, K.L., and L. Browne. (1996). 'Cultural Values and Caregiving Patterns among Asian and Pacific Islander Americans.' Unpublished paper, School of Social Work, University of Hawaii, Honolulu. A review of literature and research in Hawaii related to the caregiving patterns to the elderly among the multiethnic groups living in Hawaii.

Glezer, H. (1991). 'Support and Care between Generations.' *Family Matters* (Australia) 30, 44–6. What kind of reciprocity is there among the generations in Australia?

Koopman-Boyden, P.G., ed. (1993). *New Zealand's Aging Society: The Implications.* Wellington: Daphne Brussell Associates. A good collection of papers on seniors in New Zealand, including Maori society.

Martin, L. (1990). 'Changing Intergenerational Family Relations in East Asia.' *Annals* 510 (July), 102–14. Changing generational relations in selected countries in East Asia.

Ming-Kwan, L. (1988). 'Family and Social Life.' In Lau Siu-Kai et al., eds. *Indicators of Social Development: Hong Kong.* Hong Kong: Chinese University Press. A study of changing family life in Hong Kong, including the situations of elders in the family.

Ogawa, N., and R.D. Retherford. (1993). 'Care of the Elderly in Japan: Changing Norms and Expectations.' *Journal of Marriage and the Family* 55, 585–97. This article analyses changes in the norm of filial care for elderly parents in Japan.

Index